To Jurate Murphy, whose warm smile, twinkling eyes, and big heart has brought joy and comfort to thousands of patients.

— *Allan Zullo*

To my girls in Shropshire, Lauren and Anwen.

— *Martha Moffett*

Acknowledgments

We want to thank all the good-natured doctors, nurses, and other members of the medical profession who took the time to share with us their favorite zany but true stories.
We learned of their accounts through letters, personal interviews, E-mail, and the Internet.

A special thanks goes to Dr. John Cocker for his cooperation and especially his great sense of humor. As publisher of *Stitches, The Journal of Medical Humor,* Dr. Cocker, of Newmarket, Ontario, was kind enough to allow us to recount several funny Canadian medical moments which first appeared in his delightful monthly magazine.

Douglas Fletcher, publisher of the rib-tickling *Journal of Nursing Jocularity,* deserves our gratitude as well. He shared with us some of the funniest anecdotes that have run in his much-appreciated quarterly humor magazine for nurses.

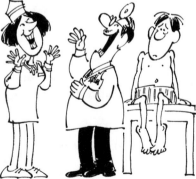

We also are grateful to *Medical Economics*, which granted us permission to reprint items from its humorous regular feature "In the Jocular Vein."

Finally, we want to thank *Readers Digest* for letting us reprint several items which had been published in earlier issues.

Contents

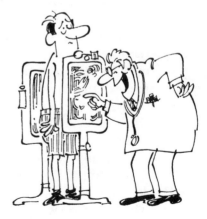

The Admitting Office

Welcome to the zany world of medicine!

Zany? But isn't medicine a somber world of pain, illness, and death? Of AIDS, SIDS, and STD? Of diseases named Alzheimer's, Chron's, and Lyme? Yes. But it is also a world of comfort, recovery, and birth. Of caring, compassion, and charity—and comedy.

You can find sick humor most anywhere—in the ER and the OR, in the waiting room and the examining room, in the pediatrics ward and the psychiatric ward.

This book celebrates the outrageous moments that have blessed doctors, nurses, and medical staff with memories that brought each a smile wider than a surgical mask. They're not likely to forget such persons as:

* The man who went to the doctor with an embarrassing bed-wetting problem, only to discover later that it was caused by a leak in his water bed.

* The patient who kept mistakenly using his oral medication as suppositories.

* The victim of chest pain who figured that since she was paying for an emergency room visit, the doctor might as well examine her hemorrhoids.

* The fisherman who needed a hook removed from his scrotum.

* The two alcoholics who fought over the color of the elephants they saw dancing in the hospital corridor.

Amid the pain and suffering they see every day, physicians relish those special moments when they must fight to keep a straight face after dealing with:

* The patient who felt better inserting suppositories still wrapped in foil rather than unwrapped ones.

* The husband who offered the doctor twice his fee not to cure his wife's laryngitis.

* The mother who chewed out the doctor for giving her daughter birth control pills without the mother's permission—even though the daughter was thirty-six years old.

Patients aren't the only ones who can lighten up an examining room. Doctors can too—with their own goofs and gaffes such as:

* The tired gynecologist who absentmindedly told his stirruped patient, "Say aah."

* Another OB-GYN man who inadvertently mixed up his words and told a skittish new patient to wait while he got undressed.

* The physician who wrote on a patient's chart, "A pelvic examination was done on the floor."

* The intern who noted that "the patient was unresponsive in bed."

These delightful incidents are gems in a tense, serious world of life and death. Doctors, nurses, and others in the medical profession know all about grief and heartache. They see it and feel it every day. But they also know how essential laughter is—for themselves and their patients. Laughter is a great healer.

So go ahead and read *Sick Humor*—just for the health of it.

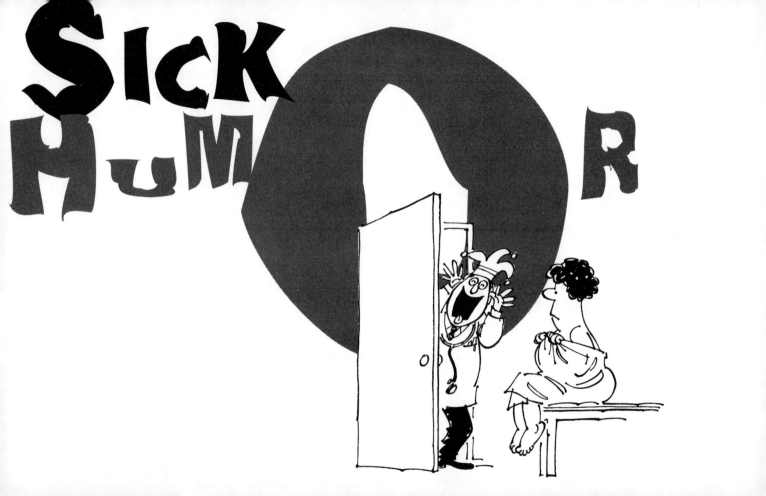

The Examining Room

Blind Man's Bluff

Dr. June T. Martin of Pittsfield, Massachusetts, had a male patient who needed a barium enema exam.

An X-ray technologist led him into a room where a hospital gown was laid out near the head of a bed. "I'll wait for you at the end of the hall," she said. Pointing to the gown, she instructed, "Take off your clothes and put that on over your head."

After several minutes went by, the technologist became concerned when the man failed to appear. She went back into the room and couldn't believe her eyes. There was the man, stark naked, with a pillowcase covering his head, groping his way along the wall!

Trial and Error

An encounter with a patient who suffered from nonspecific pruritus—itching—led Dr. Marvin D. Abrams of Vineland, New Jersey, to word his instructions more carefully.

He had advised her to "try" the remedy he prescribed four times a day for a week and then let him know the results.

Soon after leaving the office, the patient returned and handed the receptionist the prescription torn in half. "Tell Dr. Abrams to try this medicine himself," she said curtly. "If he finds that it works, then I'll use it."

Talk about Compliance!

Dr. Carl E. Couch of Garland, Texas, performed a physical on a twelve-year-old boy who was trying out for his school's football team. During the examination, the boy's mother was in the room with him and the doctor.

When Dr. Couch was ready to do a genital exam and check for a hernia, he said to the mother, "Why don't you just turn your back for a moment while I examine him."

She immediately did what she was told and turned to face the wall.

Dr. Couch then told the boy, "Now just slip off your slacks."

To the physician's shock, he looked up to see the mother worriedly gazing over her shoulder as she dropped her pants.

Myopic in More Ways Than One

A twenty-two-year-old female college student came to Dr. Joseph S. Neigut of San Antonio, Texas, for a contact lens fitting.

Dr. Neigut placed lenses on her eyes and then projected a letter chart on the wall twenty feet away. "Go as low as you can go," he asked her.

To his bemusement, she slid down and out of the chair.

Hitting the Bottle

After diagnosing an ear infection in a baby, an intern gave the child's mother a bottle of a pink antibiotic suspension as well as a bottle of vitamin drops. He also went over the instructions very carefully so she knew how to administer the medications.

The mother brought her baby back in a week for a checkup. An examination revealed that the baby was doing fine.

"Continue the medication until it is gone," the intern told the mother.

"I have plenty of drops left but no more of the pink medicine," she said.

"But the suspension should have lasted for at least ten days. Just exactly how have you been administering the medicine?"

"Well, I put the drops in her ear every day. But she drank the whole bottle of pink medicine from her baby bottle on the very first day."

Don't wake him up. He's got insomnia. He's trying to sleep it off.

— Chico Marx, *comedian*

Hard to Swallow

When Dr. Larry Rubens of Petoskey, Michigan, was in his junior year of medical school, he had an internal medicine rotation at the local Veterans Administration Hospital.

One of his patients was a happy old gent with white hair who had spent a long time there for evaluation of vague complaints. Upon examination, one of his ailments was obvious—he suffered from hemorrhoids.

The patient's medication regimen included the stool softener Colace to be taken orally, and Anusol suppositories. As was often the case at the VA, the medications were left at the bedside for the patients to administer to themselves.

However, this particular patient had a problem. He could never remember that Anusol was a suppository, so he would unwrap it first and then eat it. The doctors and nurses spent endless times on rounds trying to properly instruct the patient. He tried his best to do the right thing, but he just couldn't remember what that was. He ate lots and lots of Anusol.

One day, Rubens came into his room. The patient was beaming from ear to ear, obviously proud of himself. He said, "Doc, watch me. I've got it now!" That said, he picked up a Colace capsule and started to put it into his mouth. He looked at it, hesitated, and then in one swift move, crammed it right up his rectum!

Foiled Again!

A female patient was sent to Dr. A.L. Russell of Bramalea, Ontario, for severe migraine attacks. After trying every known oral medication without success, she agreed to try ergotamine-containing suppositories. Dr. Russell went through the normal advice regarding the insertion and warned of possible side effects such as nausea and diarrhea.

Two weeks later, the patient, looking radiant and happy, announced that the suppositories had worked wonders. There was only one minor problem. She complained that the sharpness of the suppositories occasionally caused a little rectal irritation when she inserted them. Dr. Russell realized that his patient was using the suppositories with the foil covering still on. Diplomatically, he suggested that she try the suppositories without the foil.

The patient returned two weeks later, looking haggard and tired. The suppositories caused nausea and vomiting, which made her headaches worse. She told Dr. Russell in no uncertain terms that she was going back to her original method of insertion without removing the foil.

Recalled Dr. Russell, "I must admit that every time I wrote a repeat prescription, I had an uneasy feeling. [However], I felt, after a great deal of soul-searching, that it wouldn't be in the patient's best interest to destroy this powerful placebo effect."

A Long Walk to the Ocean

When Dr. Roger Butler of St. John's, Newfoundland, began his practice in a small hospital, he felt he possessed firm communication skills and a natural ability to relate to his fellow Newfoundlanders.

One day, the head nurse directed him into the treatment room where he faced a poverty-stricken eighty-year-old female patient suffering from the ravages of an acute case of piles. Dr. Butler suggested she go home and bathe three times a day in salt water.

After the doctor left the room, the head nurse, noticing the patient was troubled, asked, "Is something the matter?"

Replied the woman, "Does Dr. Butler know I live three miles from the salt water?"

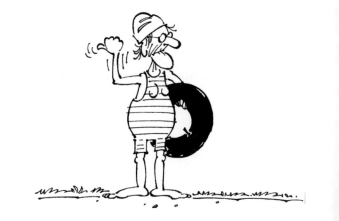

The Color Purple

Dr. Rita A. Mariotti of Woodbury Heights, New Jersey, shared the following story:

Puzzled by the odd purplish appearance of a young woman's vaginal discharge, a resident asked if she was using a vaginal medication.

"Not really," replied the patient, "only jelly, like the doctor told me when he fitted my diaphragm. He said any kind of jelly would do, and all I had in the house was grape."

Turning to Prayer

While a medical student was examining a very slender, flat-chested young woman, Dr. Thomas G. Del Giorno Jr. of Philadelphia talked to the patient.

"Do you check yourself regularly for breast masses?" he asked.

The woman instantly replied, "I *pray* for breast masses."

I enjoy convalescence. It is the part that makes the illness worthwhile.

— George Bernard Shaw, *Irish playwright*

Lady of the Night

Dr. M.D. Makin of Vanderhoof, British Columbia, was once a resident on call in a busy teaching hospital in Durban when the entire emergency room staff burst out laughing one night at 2 A.M. He soon found out why.

An intern had examined a slightly weary woman who suffered from a fairly severe vaginal discharge. He diagnosed the problem as gonorrhea. Not realizing his patient was a prostitute, the intern innocently suggested that the woman send her husband in later that morning to be treated as well.

"I'm not married," she said.

"Well, then, send your boyfriend in for treatment," the intern told her.

"I don't have a boyfriend," she replied.

Somewhat exasperated, the naive intern suggested, "Whoever you think gave you this disease should come in for treatment."

She looked him in the eye and said, "Doctor, when you eat a tin of beans, do you know which bean it is that makes you fart?"

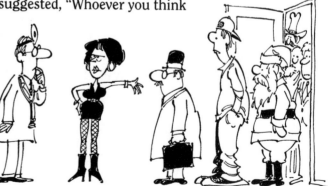

Perpetual Emotion

A young man who recently got married sounded bewildered and desperate when he confided to Dr. John D. Rosen that he was having a problem getting an erection. The patient feared he couldn't satisfy his wife.

The doctor gave him an injection with assurance that it would help him overcome his difficulty. A few weeks later, Dr. Rosen of Corona del Mar, California, saw the patient again.

"So, did the shot work?" asked the doctor.

"At first, it worked great," the groom replied. "The first night was terrific. On Saturday and Sunday, everything still went fine in the morning and afternoon and night, and also Monday morning and lunchtime. But then, that evening, the same darn problem!"

Vile Buddies

After a patient had recovered from a heart attack, he and his wife went to the office of Dr. Jerome J. Schneyer of Southfield, Michigan.

The physician explained in detail the importance of diet and exercise, and that smoking was definitely out of the question. He added that if the patient took care of himself he could lead a fulfilling, active life.

"That's all well and good," interrupted the man's wife. "But you better tell my husband this five and six times a week stuff has to stop."

Dr. Schneyer told her not to be concerned. He pointed out that, according to medical studies, sex after a heart attack can actually be beneficial.

She was hardly thrilled by the news. "You men!" she snapped. "You're all alike!"

The Truth Will Out

A sixteen-year-old patient signed himself in at the office of Dr. James Holder of Brooklyn. On a form required of new patients, the young man looked at the list of medical complaints and checked off "Penile Drainage" and "Burning with Urination."

Under "Responsible Party," he listed his girlfriend's name.

Fore Score

A recently married teenage girl visited Dr. R.C. Full of Marseilles, Illinois, complaining that sex with her husband wasn't as pleasant as she had expected.

"It's all over in five or six minutes," she lamented. A thoughtful look crossed her face as she added, "Maybe we don't engage in enough foul play."

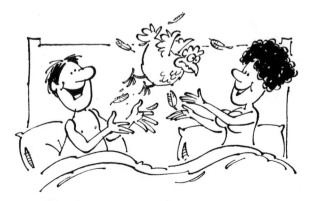

Maybe This Question Needs Refining

Dr. Jeffery J. Rabinovitz of Placerville, California, recalled the time when a family practitioner he knew was doing a routine physical on one of his adolescent patients.

As was his custom, the doctor asked the teenager whether he was sexually active.

"Uh, yes I am," came the reply.

"Well, are you using any protection?" asked the doctor.

"Oh," said the teen, "you mean active with someone else!"

Cost-Consciousness

Based on a referral from Dr. Robert W. Begley of Anderson, Indiana, a patient with bleeding hemorrhoids visited a proctologist.

During the examination, the proctologist was in the midst of inserting a sigmoidoscope when the patient asked, "Say, Doc, how much does that instrument cost?"

Finding that an odd question at that particular moment, the proctologist responded, "Why do you want to know?"

"Well," said the grimacing patient, "if it's going to hurt as much coming out as it did going in, I'll buy it and leave it there."

Fame Game

Dr. Ronald G. Worland of Medford, Oregon, reported that one of his colleagues wanted a patient to consult an ophthalmologist.

The doctor suggested one particular specialist, but the patient shook her head. "I don't care to go to a doctor who advertises," she explained.

The physician then made another recommendation. But once again, she declined, saying, "He advertises too."

The doctor thought a moment and then came up with a third name. "I don't want to see him either," she stated.

"Why not?" asked the now exasperated doctor.

"Because," she answered, "I never heard of him."

The Bright Side of Dialysis

There is at least one advantage of being a chronic hemodialysis patient.

It came to light one Monday morning when Ed, a patient of Dr. Richard A. Sherman of New Brunswick, New Jersey, showed up for a treatment. Ed, a heavyset thirty-four-year-old, had gained more weight than usual over the weekend, resulting in a difficult treatment.

As Ed was completing his dialysis, Dr. Sherman asked Ed about the weight gain. "It was worth the discomfort today," said Ed. Then he explained that he had won a sizable wager at a bar the previous Saturday night.

The bet? Who could drink the most beer without having to relieve himself.

Going Too Far

According to Dr. Joseph D. Wassersug of Braintree, Massachusetts, a surgeon friend of his performed a biopsy on an elderly man.

Later, with the man and his daughter sitting in the office, the doctor broke the bad news: He had found cancer.

The patient's daughter was furious. She ranted and raved and threatened to sue for malpractice. "My father gave you permission only for a biopsy," she claimed. "He never gave you permission to find any cancer!"

He Slept on It

A thirty-nine-year-old patient of Dr. Alan Searle of Port Orchard, Washington, was alarmed about his sudden and unexpected problem of bed-wetting.

After an examination revealed that the patient appeared to be in excellent health, Dr. Searle scheduled a urological consultation. To his surprise, Dr. Searle soon learned that the patient had canceled the consultation appointment, telling the receptionist that the problem had been resolved.

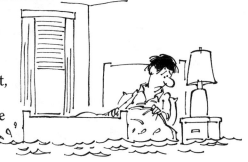

Months later, when the patient returned with a different complaint, Dr. Searle asked if he had any further bed-wetting episodes.

"Nope," replied the patient with a grin, "not since we fixed the hole in the water bed."

Auto Suggestion

Dr. James Wilson of Hampton, Virginia, recalled the time when a colleague of his tried to calm a young man slated for orthopedic surgery.

The doctor told the patient that the anesthetic would put him to sleep during the procedure. "It's as safe as driving a car," said the doctor, reassuringly.

"Oh, yeah?" replied the patient. "That's why I'm here."

Catch of the Dazed

Dr. S.D. Madduri of Poplar Bluff, Missouri, was the emergency room physician in a small rural hospital when a woman brought in her husband with a fish hook caught in the crotch of his pants. The poor man was in pain, and no wonder. The eye of the hook was penetrating his scrotum.

It took forty-five minutes for Dr. Madduri to carefully remove the hook. The doctor then went to the waiting room and told the patient's wife that her husband would be fine. Curious, Dr. Madduri asked, "What happened?"

"Well, Doc," she replied with a pronounced Missouri accent, "we were fishing on the river when Tom's line got caught on a tree limb over the water,

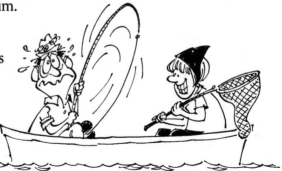

and he yanked it real hard. It bounced back and got him in the crotch." She hesitated for a moment and then added with a smile, "It looks like we got the catch of the day!"

Getting Bowled Over

Tired of the hospital and eager to return to her family, a female patient pleaded with Dr. John W. Tyznik to discharge her.

Even though she hadn't fully recovered from pancreatitis, Dr. Tyznik, of Gahanna, Ohio, reluctantly consented. But he strongly advised her to get bed rest, eat a special diet, and come for a follow-up visit the next day.

Later that evening, Dr. Tyznik received a call from his answering service: "Your patient thinks she was sent home too soon. She's weak and nauseated and wants to talk to you."

The doctor felt like kicking himself for allowing his patient to talk him into granting an early discharge. But he quickly changed his mind when the answering service added, "She wants you to page her at the bowling alley."

Anybody who goes to see a psychiatrist ought to have his head examined.

—Samuel Goldwyn, *movie producer*

It's as Simple as Your CBAs

When Dr. Patrick Taylor of Vancouver, British Columbia, was in his final year of medical school, he worked with a family physician.

One day, six-year-old Alexander, who had been a thorn in the side of his teacher and his doctor, came for an examination, which Dr. Taylor observed. The boy's mother wanted to enlist the weight of the doctor's opinion in her continuing battle with the school.

The teacher told the mother that she suspected Alexander's unruly behavior and his performance in class came from the fact that he was dyslexic. This was a terrible insult to the mother.

The family doctor was trying to be as sympathetic as possible, a task rendered all the harder by Alexander's efforts to hit his younger brother in the examining room. Any suggestion that her little darling had a problem was met with extreme resistance.

The doctor tried to explain that dyslexia was a difficulty with the written word, often characterized by an inability to read letters in the correct sequence. But the mother interrupted him.

"What do you mean, can't read?" she snapped. "My Alexander knows his ABCs backward!"

Moving Metaphors

During the days when Dr. T.R. Aitken of Stratford, Ontario, had a small-town general practice in New Zealand in the early 1980s, he saw his share of colorful characters.

One evening, he received a call from a farmer's wife who was concerned about her husband. The man had a problem with pain from constipation, and had been consuming copious quantities of Tylenol with codeine.

"He hasn't had a bowel motion in ten days," she told Dr. Aitken. "This morning he took Epsom salts."

"What was the outcome?" asked the doctor.

"Now he has no control of his bowels whatsoever."

The doctor soon examined the farmer and gave him a prescription for a fleet enema. Then Dr. Aitken made arrangements for him to be catheterized at the nearby hospital because he had gone into urinary retention.

Upon seeing the patient the next day, Dr. Aitken asked, "How have things worked out?"

"Doctor," replied the farmer, "you moved a mountain and diverted a river."

No Nude's Good News

Dr. Philip R. Alper of Burlingame, California, treated a seventy-eight-year-old patient named Victor for prostatitis and then billed Medicare accordingly.

Mystifyingly, Medicare wrote back, asking whether Victor was male or female. Dr. Alper's secretary answered that even if Victor's name wasn't a clue to his sex, the diagnosis certainly was. Incredibly, the secretary's letter did little good. After three months, the claim was still unpaid.

So Victor took matters into his own hands. He wrote to Medicare and threatened to send a nude photo—a frontal view of himself—to prove that he was a male.

In no time at all, Medicare sent the check.

Better Late than Never
Dr. Michael S. Niziol of Dryden, New York, treated a patient who came in with acute chest pain.

During history-taking, the patient sheepishly admitted that despite the doctor's previous warnings, he hadn't stopped smoking. Shortly after his admission, the electrocardiogram confirmed that he had acute ischemia, limited blood flow because of a clogged or blocked blood vessel.

Dr. Niziol explained to him that he was having a heart attack and required immediate admission to one of the three hospitals in the area.

"Do you have a preference?" asked the doctor.

The patient looked him straight in the eye and said, "Yes, I'll take nonsmoking."

Not on Good Footing
Julie Monturo of Newark, Ohio, was barefoot one day when she was retrieving some items from her cellar. Unfortunately, she stepped on a nail.

Julie promptly called her physician and went in for a tetanus shot.

Two months later, she was barefoot once more when she cut her toe while raking. A slight infection set in, so she returned to her doctor for treatment.

This time, attached to a prescription for antibiotics was a second prescription: "Wear shoes."

Fingering The Blame

A man was getting his mandatory physical examination for an Australian visa from a young, attractive female physician.

Since he was about fifteen years older than she was, he felt at liberty to have a little fun with the exam. "Am I gonna die today, Doc?" he asked while she listened to his heart.

"Do you find me unnervingly attractive?" he queried as she felt his paunch.

The doctor played it straight and went about the examination in a professional manner. He couldn't tell what was going on in her mind; whether or not she thought he was a jerk or a chauvinist. He simply couldn't read her.

Then she put latex over her finger and greased it up with K-Y Jelly. Suddenly, the old boy had a change of face. "Oh, no, you're not gonna do that, are you? Why don't we skip that part? We'll just go ahead and say that you did it and that everything was fine."

"Drop your pants and bend over," she ordered.

Trying to joke his way out of the situation he asked, "Shouldn't you have somebody else in the room before you do this?"

He watched her face very closely and thought he saw a hint of a smile when she snapped back, "We'll get the whole office in here if it'll make you feel better."

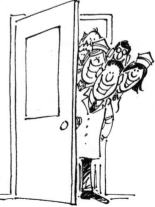

Is That in the Bible?

Registered nurse Mitch Mason of Plantation, Florida, helped treat a man who was brought into the trauma room after being struck by a car. The patient suffered compound fractures of both legs.

Upon his arrival, the doctor asked him, "What happened?"

The patient looked up at the physician and said, "God moves in mysterious ways—and sometimes He moves like a Chevrolet."

Seeing Eye-to-Eye

Optometrist Jeff Palmer from Middletown, Connecticut, once had a woman patient who passed an eye exam with flying colors.

"Good news," he said. "Your vision is better than normal. It's 20/15."

Instead of being pleased, the patient seemed quite perturbed and declared, loud enough for all in the full waiting room to hear, "Hey, I paid for 20/20. I want 20/20!"

I "No" How You Feel

Registered nurse Amy Luckowski was taking care of a confused surgical patient one night in the ICU. After running through all the usual orientation questions, she asked him what her name was.

He growled, "No!"

"No?" Amy asked.

He caustically replied, "No is your name. No! You can't do this. No! You can't do that. No! You can't get out of bed. No! You can't eat."

Amy laughed and told him that was a good joke and she couldn't wait to tell her husband.

Snapped the patient, "Honey, your husband knew your name was No an hour after you got married!"

Manic Mutt

As a psychiatric nurse, Mark Darby of Omaha, Nebraska, knows that when manic-depressives are in the manic phase, they can be very upbeat and pleasant—and quite funny.

Janet was one such patient. She liked to yell for her nurse rather than use the call light. Darby and the other nurses tended to ignore her behavior in hopes she would stop doing it.

Darby was assigned to Janet one day when she was very manic. When Janet saw Darby standing at the other end of a long hall, she began calling his name. When he ignored her, she continued to repeat it faster and louder as she walked down the hall toward him.

Janet was screaming, "Mark! Mark! Mark! Mark! Mark!" She walked right up to him, looked him in the eye and kept repeating his name. Janet suddenly stopped and said, "Gee, that sounds like a harelipped dog."

Sticking It to Him

In a North Carolina county, an "ambulance junkie" was well known to the local emergency medical technicians. Every time he got bored, he would fake an emergency and call the ambulance.

The EMTs got tired of his antics and so did the county, which was picking up the tab for the emergency rides. So they came up with a plan that ended his joyrides.

The next time the medics received one of his calls, they zoomed out to his home and loaded him into the ambulance. On the way to the hospital, an EMT pulled out a huge needle and told him that they would need to use it on him. He hasn't called since.

Just Another Day in the Psychiatry Wing

One evening while Dr. Karen Nepveu was doing the psychiatry rotation in medical school, she was called to the emergency room to evaluate a man for possible admission.

During the mental-status exam, Dr. Nepveu, of Montague, Massachusetts, asked the standard question, "Have you been hearing voices?"

"Oh, no," he stated firmly. He paused slightly before his face revealed a look of surprise. Then he told Dr. Nepveu, "Wait! There's one now. It said 'liar.'"

Nerve-Wracking

Dr. Harry B. Andrews of Fremont, California, was signing out a male patient after treatment for one of his repeated bouts of overdosing on tranquilizers.

The doctor was trying to be understanding, but it wasn't easy. Not after the patient, who was still weaving unsteadily, said in a slurred voice, "Doc, before I go, can you give me something for my nerves?"

Stool Pigeon

An intern was called in to take the medical history of a patient. He was admitted into the hospital complaining of chest and abdominal pain after smoking crack.

As part of the history, the diligent medical student asked the patient, "What color is your stool?"

He gave her a funny look and replied, "White."

The student was surprised by his answer. "Are you sure?"

"Yes," he insisted. "It's been white all my life. Aren't they all white?"

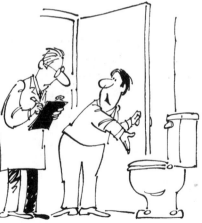

Flight Beer

At a large British teaching hospital, an alcoholic was admitted for treatment.

While making his rounds, the doctor asked the patient how he was feeling. According to Dr. Neil Carmichael of Newcastle under Lyme, England, the patient replied, "I must be missing the booze more than I had expected, Doc. When I looked out the window, I thought I saw beer cans flying past."

Just then the doctor looked up and caught a glimpse of a beer can falling past the window. He did a little investigating—and found a patient on the floor above had a secret supply of beer hidden in his room. The upstairs patient had disposed of the empties by tossing them out of the window.

Bug-Eyed

One day, during John Capps's internship at a Veterans Administration Hospital, he was doing rounds with his team when they visited a patient who had been admitted the day before with chronic obstructive pulmonary disease.

The attending physician decided to use the case to expound upon the acute neurological complications of dipsomania and managed to convince the interns that this unsuspecting fellow was about to go into the DTs.

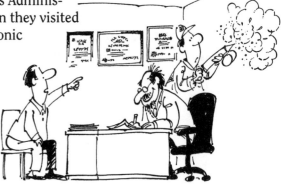

According to Dr. Capps of Gastonia, North Carolina, the attending physician started asking the usual DT-searching questions of the patient, including, "Are you seeing any bugs or insects?"

"Sure am," the patient replied, pointing to the far corner of the room.

The physician seemed pleased with the response and launched into a monologue to the interns about the nature of visual hallucinations in DTs. But then one of the medical students turned around and announced that indeed there was a sizable roach crawling up the far wall.

Needless to say, the patient did not require any Librium during his stay at the VA. But because Dr. Capps couldn't help but laugh out loud when they all spotted the roach, the attending physician made note of the intern's "unprofessional tendencies at bedside presentations" in his eventual review.

* * *

According to registered nurse Bruce Tretbar, an emergency room nurse was dealing with a man going through DTs.

Trying to find a vein for an IV, she started patting his forearm. The patient nodded, said, "Yeah, honey, I see them too," and started swatting at his arm.

Too Close for (Southern) Comfort

One night while registered nurse Mitch Mason was on duty, two well-intoxicated patients were kept near the nurse's desk because both were having DTs and warranted close observation. The patients were placed close to each other in the hall.

That turned out to be a mistake.

The two began to fight over the true color of the elephants they both saw dancing in the hall.

While I'm Here . . .

Dr. Sunita Puri of Decatur, Alabama, examined a woman who was brought into the emergency room, complaining of chest pains.

After the physician treated her aggressively and made her comfortable, the pain disappeared. Dr. Puri then ordered some blood tests and X-rays.

While they waited for the results, the woman grew impatient. Finally she told the doctor, "Since I'm paying for this expensive examining room, I want to have my hemorrhoids checked."

Good Luck Collecting that Debt

No response to a billing inquiry has ever topped a note a patient sent to Dr. Mary O. Anderson of Leonidas, Michigan.

It read: "I hope to pay up after I get back to work if I find a job and my wife and girlfriend have their babies and I get my truck fixed. That is, if I'm not in jail on the income tax charge."

Bill of Complaint

The office manager of Dr. Lawrence S. Slotnick of Greensboro, North Carolina, asked a patient if the doctor had given him a clean bill of health.

The patient's companion spoke up, "He gives you a bill whether you're healthy or not."

A Phone of Contention

During office hours, a repairman came in to check the intermittent but persistent problems that Dr. Marie T. Kelly was having with a new telephone system.

Dr. Kelly of Fort Worth, Texas, bristled when the man suggested that perhaps she wasn't dialing properly. She fumed even more after he left.

As she walked into the adjacent examining room, Dr. Kelly received a steely glance from an elderly patient who had been waiting there. "I trusted my life to you when you operated on me," said the patient, "and now I find you don't even know how to dial a telephone!"

The best cure for hypochondria is to forget about your body and get interested in somebody else's.

— Goodman Ace, *humorist*

Beyond Recall

A distraught patient called the home of Dr. Edwin E. Buckner of Longview, Texas, saying she needed his immediate attention.

The physician's wife told her he was out, but he would get in touch with her soon if she would leave her phone number.

"Oh, I couldn't do that," said the patient. "My number is unlisted and I never give it out."

* * *

One night, pediatrician Joseph F.J. Curi of Torrington, Connecticut, received an urgent nighttime call at home from the mother of a patient.

"Doctor, my daughter came home from school today with head lice," she explained. "I used Kwell shampoo on her, my husband, and myself. Should I also use it on our cat?"

Although he was annoyed that she had called so late in the evening with such a question, Dr. Curi kept his cool. He answered her by saying, "Why don't you call your veterinarian?"

Her voice registered shock as she said, "What? At this hour?"

Would you please turn on the television. I'd like to see if I'm still alive and how I'm doing.

— Murray Haydon, *artificial heart recipient*

What a Bite

Although Nancy Bishop's grandfather had undergone extensive dental work, he was nonetheless appalled by the amount of his bill.

He talked to the dentist, who defended the bill by saying, "I've had years of expensive schooling, and when you require my services, you must be prepared to pay for that schooling."

Grandpa mused this over for a moment and then asked, "All by myself?"

* * *

The dentistry patients of Dr. Michael M. Stryker of San Antonio, Texas, are called and reminded the day before their scheduled appointments.

During an office visit, a businessman was in an especially good humor and explained why. "My staff kids me about the high opinion I have of myself," he told Dr. Stryker. "Yesterday your receptionist left a message that had them in stitches."

He then revealed the contents of the memo his secretary had handed him: "Your crown is ready."

* * *

A longtime patient arrived at the office of dentist Gerald B. Berenson of Shrewsbury, Massachusetts.

She claimed she had a one o'clock appointment, but the receptionist said the patient's name was not anywhere in the scheduling book. The woman insisted that someone had called her to say that it was time for her yearly examination and cleaning and had set up the appointment.

The receptionist told her that the dentist always sent out reminders to all his patients before his office staff calls to arrange a time. The woman was miffed by what she heard and left in a huff.

However, within an hour, the patient phoned Dr. Berenson's office to apologize. Then, sheepishly, she told the receptionist that when she returned home, she found a man waiting patiently on her front steps. He was from the oil company and had come to give her furnace its yearly examination and cleaning.

Harmed Services

At a base hospital in Cherry Point, North Carolina, a Marine Corps warrant officer was trying unsuccessfully to get the medical personnel to issue him new eyeglasses without an appointment.

Just then, a two-star general came into the room, and the warrant officer snapped sharply to attention, greeting the top brass, "Good morning, Colonel!"

"Mister," snarled the general, "if you can't tell a two-star general from a colonel, you better get glasses."

The warrant officer didn't have to wait for an appointment.

* * *

One night, army doctor Tim O'Connor of Columbia, Missouri, was taking his turn in the emergency room of the base hospital at Fort Leonard Wood. A young recruit was brought in with a high fever and abdominal pain.

Dr. O'Connor suspected the new soldier was suffering from appendicitis. Pressing on the young man's abdomen, the physician asked, "Does this hurt?"

"Yes, sir," he moaned through clenched teeth.

Then Dr. O'Connor examined the area where the appendix is located. "How about here?"

To the doctor's surprise, the recruit replied, "No."

"No?" echoed the doctor.

"I mean," stammered the recruit, "NO, SIR!"

My doctor gave me six months to live. But when I couldn't pay the bill, he gave me six months more.

— Henny Youngmen, *comedian*

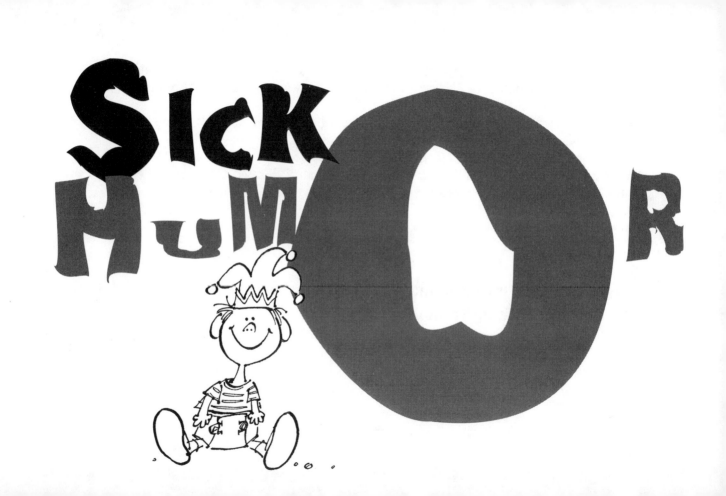

The Pediatric Ward

Not the Lesson He Expected

Dr. Gil Solomon's four-year-old daughter was so curious that she somehow got a rock stuck up her nose.

Dr. Solomon of West Hills, California, tried closing the other nostril and blowing through her mouth to dislodge the rock. Only nasal secretions came out.

He took his daughter to the emergency room where an otolaryngologist was called in. "This is no small rock," he said, after examining the little girl. After a few delicate maneuvers, he managed to dislodge the rock.

As Dr. Solomon was leaving the ER, he turned to his daughter and said, "I hope you learned something from this."

"I did, Daddy," she declared. "Next time I stick a rock up my nose, I won't push it in so far."

Error of Omission

While at home on call one day, Dr. Thomas Slayton of Flossmoor, Illinois, was getting annoyed because his pager kept going off so often. Each time that it did, he muttered a mild swear word, although he was barely aware he was doing so. However, others in the household definitely were aware.

The following week, when he was once again at home on call, the pager beeped. This time, Dr. Slayton answered the page without a trace of irritation.

His two-and-a-half-year-old daughter shot him a puzzled look and said, "Daddy, you forgot to say 'damn it!'"

Not the Shirt Off My Back

As a way to help her pediatric patients relate to a female physician, Dr. Kathleen M. Holland of Kerrville, Texas, tries to maintain a relaxed attitude.

One day, she encouraged a three-year-old boy to watch as she examined his older brother. After the examination, Dr. Holland let the little boy slip her stethoscope from her neck. He walked around the room, listening to the wall and other silent objects.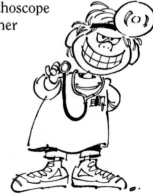

Then he returned to the doctor. "I want to listen to you," he said.

"Okay," replied Dr. Holland, grinning at his mother.

Holding the stethoscope in the proper position, the little boy unhesitatingly commanded, "Take off your shirt."

The "examination" came to a quick end.

On Close Examination

Dr. William Keenan of St. Louis noticed how enthralled his four-year-old patient seemed with him. The physician couldn't quite understand why the boy kept staring so intently at him.

When the boy's mother remarked on his fascinated gaze, the little tyke exclaimed, "Yeah, Mom! He has more hair in his nose than anyone I ever saw!"

How about Oil and Vinegar?

Dr. Paul Collins of Wichita Falls, Texas, accompanied a seven-year-old boy to the emergency room to repair a serious laceration from a bicycle accident.

The young patient was understandably apprehensive during the whole procedure, so Dr. Collins calmly explained what he was doing before each step. When he was finished, the physician announced, "Now all we have to do is apply the dressing."

The boy held up his hands and declared, "Anything but Roquefort. I hate that!"

Tough Act to Follow

Dr. Adele Engelberg of New York was examining a cute four-year-old girl who had won her heart.

"Do you know who is my favorite doctor in the whole world?" the little patient asked.

Glowing in anticipation, Dr. Engelberg replied, "No. Who?"

Announced the girl, "The doctor who was here before you."

Set 'em Up!

An eight-year-old boy accompanied his mother to the office of Dr. G.M. Buehler of Jeffersonville, Indiana.

The boy watched intently as the nurse mixed a blood sample with solution for a white blood cell count. "Oh," he asked, "what are you making—a Bloody Mary?"

The Wonders of Science

A young boy came into the office of Dr. Richard A. Rosen of Providence, Rhode Island, for evaluation of a respiratory infection and sore throat.

Dr. Rosen called in the nurse practitioner, who took a throat culture using a cotton swab.

"What's that for?" asked the boy.

"We'll plant this in the lab and see what grows," answered the nurse.

The boy's eyes lit up with the excitement of learning something new as he exclaimed, "So *that's* how you grow new Q-tips!"

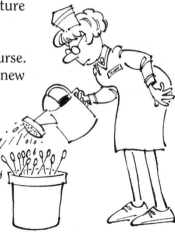

Zap! No More Doctor

In the office of Dr. Joseph P. Bark of Lexington, Kentucky, a nurse was trying to calm a frightened six-year-old boy before the physician could perform a mole biopsy.

The nurse was teaching the teary-eyed youngster how to use the handheld control for the electric table. "This button makes the table go way up, and this button makes it go way down," the nurse told him.

Just then, the boy looked up as Dr. Bark entered the room. The little patient burst into tears and loudly asked the nurse, "Which button makes him go away?"

Skeletons in the Closet

When he was practicing at the Fort Monroe Army Hospital in Virginia, Dr. George B. Markle IV of Carlsbad, New Mexico, kept a skeleton hanging in a locker in his office.

The bones came in handy one day when Dr. Markle was examining an obnoxious army brat who was giving his mother and the doctor a very hard time. The physician had seen enough and warned the boy, "If you don't behave, I'll have to put you in that locker."

The threat did no good. The unruly child continued to act up, making it difficult for Dr. Markle to complete the examination. Finally, in exasperation, the doctor declared, "Okay, here you go!" Dr. Markle then flung open the locker door to reveal the creepy, grinning skeleton.

The wide-eyed youngster sat up straight and gasped as the doctor shook his head and said, "Uh-oh. I forgot to let the last one out."

Neither the boy's mother nor Dr. Markle had any further difficulty with him.

Trick Shot

On several occasions, a woman new to the area brought her ten-year-old daughter to Dr. LeRoy Bernstein of Las Vegas.

The girl complained of vague ailments. Despite thorough examinations, the doctor couldn't find any physical causes for the symptoms she described. Each time, the doctor pulled her mother aside and said the girl wasn't really sick. The woman seemed to accept grudgingly his advice for purely symptomatic treatment for her daughter.

But then one day, when the girl once again showed up at his office, Dr. Bernstein discovered that this time the girl definitely was suffering from a sore throat and probably sinusitis.

The mother felt a sense of satisfaction that since her daughter was truly sick, she should receive real medical treatment and not symptomatic care. So when Dr. Bernstein told them he was going to prescribe some oral medications, the mother bristled and asked, "No shots? Dr. Brown (the girl's previous physician) used to give her a shot every time she was sick."

That's when the girl piped up, "Yes, even when I was faking!"

Tasty Judgment

Dr. Kathleen McAuliffe gives her little patients suckers when their examinations are finished.

After one such exam, Dr. McAuliffe of Vancouver, Washington, told a four-year-old patient, "Save the sucker until after supper."

"Why?" asked the little girl.

"Because what you need before this sucker is nutrition."

The youngster shook her head. "We had that for lunch," she said. "I didn't like it."

Pulling No Punches

Clinical explanations usually appear on a standard form that Dr. Donald P. Dobson sees when he reviews malpractice claims.

However, there was an exception. Dr. Dobson of Portland, Oregon, saw a terse statement on the form that gave new meaning to the term "defensive medicine." It simply read: "Kid hit Doc. Doc hit kid."

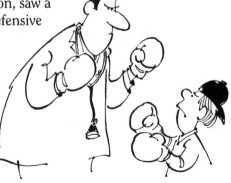

Reasonable Request

A four-year-old boy complaining of abdominal pain was brought to the emergency room.

While he waited to be examined by the doctor, the nurse came in and told the youngster, "I have to take your blood pressure."

After she did so, Dr. Alan Fuss of Omaha, Nebraska, entered the room and gave him a careful examination. Fortunately, it was not a serious problem and the physician told the boy's worried parents that he could be released for home care.

To everyone's surprise, the youngster didn't want to leave.

"I'm not going," he insisted. Then, pointing to the nurse, the boy added, "Not until she gives me back my blood pressure."

A Long Shot

Four-year-old Derek refused to give the nurse a urine sample, so Dr. Thomas J. Forristal of Cincinnati went to see him.

The doctor entered the exam room with his arm extended, holding a cup, and announced to the defiant boy, "You will put urine in this container."

Derek gave Dr. Forristal a look of astonishment and then whined, from the far corner of the room, "From here?"

That Spells "No Way"

A precocious five-year-old became a challenge for Dr. Eric J. Ruby of Taunton, Massachusetts.

The boy was in no mood for an injection that he suspected was next on the doctor's list of things to do during the examination.

Dr. Ruby was discussing immunization with the young patient's mother when the boy stood up and announced, "If DPT spells shot, I'm out of here!"

There are only two things a child will share willingly—communicable diseases and his mother's age.

— Dr. Benjamin Spock, *famed pediatrician*

Fly on the Wall

Dr. Mamta Gautam, a child psychiatrist from Ottawa, Ontario, had been treating an eight-year-old girl who had difficulty dealing with her parents' nasty divorce.

After several months of therapy, he felt she had learned to cope well with the situation. But one day her mother called Dr. Gautam. She explained that her daughter had just returned from a visit with the father and was behaving in an unbearable manner, with constant tantrums, loud arguments and other acting-out behavior.

When Dr. Gautam saw the girl in his office, she was initially sullen and refused to admit that there were any problems. He tried to coax her to tell him what she had been feeling and experiencing. She remained steadfastly quiet despite his best efforts to get her to describe the scene at home.

When all else failed, Dr. Gautam asked her, "If I were a fly on the wall in your home when you got back from your Dad's house, what would I have seen?"

"Nothing," she replied. "I'd swat you, and you'd be dead!"

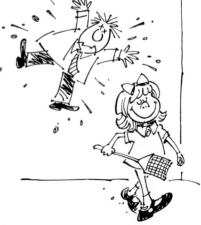

The Foreign Lesion

As a plastic surgeon, Dr. Chili Robinson of Corpus Christi, Texas, sometimes gets challenging diagnostic referrals.

On one occasion, an emergency appointment was requested for a four-year-old boy with a black lesion on his neck. His mother was sure it had not been present about a month earlier.

As he examined the robust, healthy lad, Dr. Robinson easily spotted the raised black lesion on his neck. It didn't look at all familiar. Gingerly the physician touched it—and then picked off the boy's dried chewing gum.

An Old Trick

A bright and loquacious ten-year-old girl was seeing Dr. Stanley Lofsky of Willowdale, Ontario, for a number of symptoms, including diarrhea and cramps.

The doctor felt it was appropriate to examine the stool for culture and parasites. So he explained to her the method for collecting the specimen with minimum fuss.

The method involves lifting the toilet seat and spreading plastic wrap over the bowl, then bringing down the seat while making a depression in the plastic wrap with one's fist. Once the stool is passed, and the specimen collected with the spoons provided with the sample bottle, the toilet seat is raised and the plastic wrap and remaining stool fall into the bowl and are flushed.

The young patient was listening intently, and when Dr. Lofsky got to the part about spreading plastic wrap over the bowl, she declared, "That's what I do on April Fool's Day!"

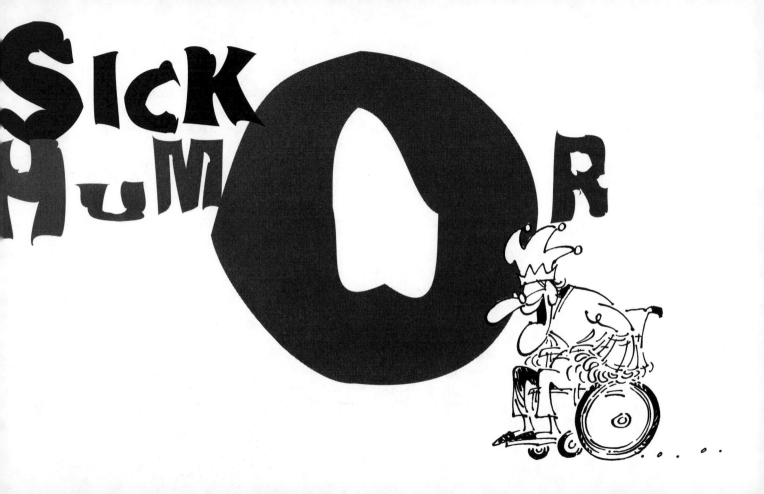

The Geriatric Ward

Sing a Different Tune

Dr. Vincent B. Pica of Trenton, New Jersey, was instilling dilating drops into an elderly patient's eyes.

"Do the drops bother you?" he asked.

"What did you say?" she responded.

Assuming she was hard of hearing, Dr. Pica inquired in a louder voice, "Do they sting?"

"Do what?" she asked, her face crinkled in an expression of not understanding.

Fighting exasperation, Dr. Pica repeated even more loudly than before, "Sting! Sting!"

To his stunned surprise, the elderly patient suddenly began warbling, "My country, 'tis of thee, sweet land of liberty . . ."

Forewarned Is Forearmed

Because of illness and vacation among his staff, Dr. Ralph H. Swerdlow of Sacramento, California, found himself alone in his office for the day.

To each female patient who had an appointment that day, he asked how she felt about being examined without being chaperoned by one of his assistants. No one had a problem.

However, there was one little, old, white-haired lady who told Dr. Swerdlow, "That doesn't bother me. But I'm taking my cane in with me just in case."

Getting an Earful

Years ago, Dr. Robert E. Falcone of Columbus, Ohio, was part of a group of interns accompanying an attending physician on morning rounds.

They entered a room where an eighty-six-year-old woman was lying impassively in bed. She made no response as the group leader greeted her. She didn't move or speak as he repeatedly inquired in an increasingly loud voice how she was feeling.

Eventually, he asked in a booming tone, "Do you have pains anywhere?"

This time, the patient reacted. "Yes," she replied with irritation dripping from her voice, "in the ear you're yelling into."

Don't Bother Fixing It

Among the favorite patients of Dr. Patricia J. Roy of Muskegon, Michigan, were a delightful elderly couple, Mel and Jean, whom she had known for a long time.

The couple often bickered and bantered back and forth with the kind of familiar affection that can only come from being married for more than forty years.

One day, Mel left a cryptic message with Dr. Roy's answering service. He said, "I'll give you twice your office-visit fee if you don't fix Jean." Perplexed by the strange offer, Dr. Roy asked her staff if they knew what Mel was talking about. One of the staff members pointed to the day's schedule of patients.

There was Jean's name for an appointment later in the day. Her complaint: "Lost my voice."

Only a Matter of Time

One day, Dr. Jerome J. Schneyer of Southfield, Michigan, was escorting a distinguished visiting medical professor on morning rounds at the hospital.

They had just left the room of an elderly alcoholic patient who had been admitted for ailments that he truly believed were terminal.

As the physicians were walking down the hall, the elderly man rushed after them. Going up to the visiting professor, the man pleaded, "Tell me the truth, Doc. How much time do I have left?"

The patient asked his question while the professor was still talking to Dr. Schneyer and didn't hear the query. Unfortunately, the professor chose that exact moment to look down at his watch. The next thing the doctors knew, the patient was lying in a dead faint on the hallway floor.

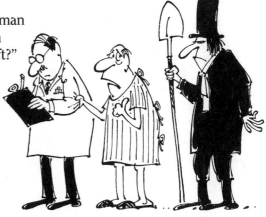

Whistling in the Dark

Dr. Vincent B. Pica of Trenton, New Jersey, was doing cataract surgery on an older woman under local anesthesia. Early in the procedure, he heard someone in the operating room whistling the hymn "Rock of Ages."

Turning with some impatience to the three nurses assisting him, Dr. Pica barked, "It's really not professional to be whistling here—especially that song."

The nurses looked at each other quizzically and denied whistling or doing anything wrong.

Then it occurred to Dr. Pica where the hymn was coming from—under the drapes. The patient herself was the one fearfully whistling "Rock of Ages."

Gender Confusion

After examining a frail, elderly patient, Dr. Christian Ulrich of Monroe, Louisiana, helped her off the examining table.

Figuring she could use help from his assistant in getting dressed, Dr. Ulrich asked the patient, "Would you like me to have Amanda come in and help you put on your clothes?"

The slightly hard of hearing patient replied, "Oh! A man! To help me put on my clothes? I'd scare him to death!"

To Tell the Truth

After examining an elderly hospital patient, Dr. Charles W. Taylor ordered an electrocardiogram as part of the workup.

Later that day, Dr. Taylor returned to the patient's room and was taken aback by the man's surly attitude.

"So, you didn't believe me when I said I was sick," the patient snapped.

"I assure you I most certainly do believe you are sick," said Dr. Taylor.

"Then why," demanded the patient, "did you have them give me a lie detector test?"

No Escape

An elderly man was referred for a postoperative radiograph following prostate surgery.

According to Dr. Randall M. Patten of Nampa, Idaho, as the patient was leaving the dressing room after the examination, an X-ray technologist discreetly pointed out to him that his fly was open.

"Don't you worry about that," replied the patient. "Ain't nothing going to be getting out of there. My urologist saw to that!"

And What Shape is That?

Dr. Anthony J. Kocalis of Chicago had just finished examining an elderly lady who had come in for a routine appointment. She was accompanied by her daughter, who listened carefully as the doctor went over the results of his examination.

As the two of them left the examining room, the patient asked her daughter, "What did the doctor say?"

"He said you were in good shape for your age," her daughter replied.

The old woman thought for a long moment and then asked, "How old am I?"

Higher Authority

Suspecting a brain tumor, Dr. M. Gerald Edelstein of Cherry Hill, New Jersey, sent a crusty old lady to a neurosurgeon who performed a spinal tap.

During the painful procedure, the obviously distressed patient looked upward and whispered, "Help me. Please help me."

The specialist tried to soothe her by saying, "I'm sorry, but I'm doing the best I can."

Raising her head, the patient gave him a chilly stare and growled, "I wasn't talking to you."

I prefer old age to the alternative.

— Maurice Chevalier, *French entertainer*

No News Is Bad News

Dr. Charles J. Wolfe of Daytona Beach, Florida, shook his head one day when a little eighty-year-old patient came in for an appointment.

Though in generally satisfactory condition for her age, she was like several of his elderly patients. She tended to be a chronic complainer. On this day, Dr. Wolfe was impressed with how fit she looked.

"So, what's troubling you today?" he asked.

"Doctor," she replied. "I've been feeling so good lately that I wanted to be checked out to see what's wrong."

Age of Consent

A gray-haired woman with a flushed face burst into the Southfield, Michigan, office of Dr. Jerome J. Schneyer while he was having a consultation with one of his female patients.

Pointing to the woman who was sitting across from the doctor, the elderly intruder glowered at Dr. Schneyer and demanded to know, "Are you giving my daughter birth control pills?"

The physician was so startled by this unexpected scene that he didn't say a word. He simply nodded.

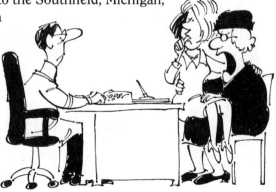

"How dare you encourage a child to do that sort of thing?" the elderly woman railed. "I'll have your license suspended!"

Finally recovering some of his composure, Dr. Schneyer told her, "Madam, that 'child' is thirty-six years old."

The woman shot him an even more hateful stare. "I'm still her mother. You should have checked with me first!"

Strange Turnabout

Though otherwise in good possession of her mental faculties, an elderly hospitalized patient was subject to nighttime confusion that bothered her roommate.

The patient was moved to another room, but her next roommate complained, too. In fact, the patient was moved four times in her first week in the hospital—from the north corridor, to the east, south, and then west.

When Dr. Frank R. Claudy of Baltimore came to see her, she was gazing pensively out the window. "You know, Doctor," she said, "this hospital is remarkable. Every seven days, it rotates a complete 360 degrees."

Aging seems to be the only available way to live a long time.

— Daniel-François-Esprit Auber, *nineteenth-century French composer*

What's a Doctor For?

For more than a year, Mrs. Jones came in for frequent visits to Dr. Saeed Mahmoodian of Bridgeport, West Virginia. The patient usually complained of a vague symptom that she blamed on old age.

Mrs. Jones wasn't a hypochondriac, however, and she had such a pleasant personality that Dr. Mahmoodian and the staff looked forward to seeing her. Then six weeks went by without a visit or even a telephone call.

When Mrs. Jones finally showed up, the doctor asked her for an explanation. Without any trace of irony, she said, "I'm sorry, Doc, I just couldn't make it in. You see, I was sick and couldn't go out anywhere."

A Mouthful of Bellyaches

Dr. Tom Campbell of Bradford, Tennessee, was called to the home of an elderly lady who said she "just wasn't feeling well."

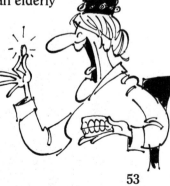

As the doctor sat listening to a list of aches, the patient's son interrupted her. "Mother," he said, "I'll give you a dime if you can name one ache you haven't had this week."

The old woman flashed a toothless grin and declared, "A toothache!" She then held out her hand and collected her dime.

Sounds Familiar

Otolaryngologist Guy Tropper, of Cornwall, Ontario, examined an elderly lady who had a cold three weeks earlier, during which developed a sensation of blockage of her ears.

Dr. Tropper readily diagnosed an ear infection, and given the recent onset, suggested simple observation. The patient seemed very disturbed by the discomfort of her blocked ears, and returned to the doctor's office two weeks later. Still complaining, she came back a third time and was more forceful, demanding the doctor "get on with it and do something about it."

"I've tried, Madam, to do what's best for you," said the physician. "And yet I have this sense that you're unhappy with what I've done so far for you."

At that very moment, her husband, who had accompanied the patient to the examining room, stood up and said, "It's funny, Doc. I've lived with her for eleven years and I still have the same feeling!"

First thing I do when I wake up in the morning is breathe on a mirror and hope it fogs.

— Early Wynn, *former major league pitcher*

Too Much Red Tape

It was one of those busy days in the admitting office at the hospital.

Several patients were filling out forms, others were being interviewed, and still more were being escorted to their rooms.

An elderly woman hesitantly entered Mildred Hays's cubicle. The woman had carefully completed her admitting forms and handed them to Mildred. At Mildred's request, the lady gave her an insurance card.

After typing in the necessary information, Mildred asked her, "What is the reason for your coming to the hospital?"

"Just to visit a friend," replied the elderly woman. "But this has taken so long, I'm not sure I have time now."

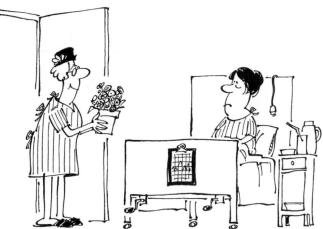

Share and Share Alike

When checking on elderly patients' lunch intake, nurse Mary Elizabeth Martucci found one woman sitting with her full tray in front of her, staring into space.

Meanwhile, her roommate was loudly enjoying her meal. When Mary asked the noneating patient why she wasn't consuming her meal, she turned and pointed to the roommate and said, "She's not done with the teeth yet."

It Was Good for Me

While on night shift in the ICU with two other nurses, registered nurse Carey Frank was concerned that a ninety-two-year-old female patient hadn't voided in some time.

The only female on duty tried to catheterize the elderly woman. But the patient was more than a little confused and not entirely cooperative. So Frank and the other male nurse were called in to help.

While one retracted the patient's knees, Frank held the flashlight and the female nurse tried to find the right opening. After about twenty minutes and nine tries, the patient exclaimed, "My goodness, I haven't done this since my husband died."

Let's Not Rush Things

Dr. John Hirsh of Fort Lauderdale performed a hysterectomy on a sixty-four-year-old woman.

Six weeks later, the doctor did a postoperative checkup of the patient while her seventy-four-year-old husband remained in the waiting room. The woman asked Dr. Hirsh when she and her husband could resume sexual intercourse.

The physician assumed his patient would be pleased when he told her, "Anytime now."

She thought for a moment and said, "Fine. I'll tell him another six weeks."

Never Too Late

At the time of his annual checkup, Dr. Arona Kagnoff of Corona del Mar, California, found the eighty-seven-year-old patient spry and alert and in exceptionally good condition for his age.

The elderly man told the doctor that his wife had recently died and then hesitantly mentioned that he had been impotent for many years. Dr. Kagnoff was surprised and asked, "Why hadn't you brought this problem to my attention before?"

"Well," said the patient. "I was married then and it didn't matter. But now I'm single again."

Old Smolders Never Die

Dr. Joseph B. Chanatry of Utica, New York, gave a complete gynecological exam to an elderly patient who had a vaginal vault prolapse—the floor of her vagina had collapsed.

He offered her two options of treatment: If she wasn't sexually active, he could do a colpectomy, thereby removing the vagina. If she was still sexually active, he could do a colpopexy and suture the prolapsed vagina to the abdominal wall, thus preserving her sexual functions.

After listening to Dr. Chanatry, the patient's married daughter, who had accompanied her to the exam, told the physician, "Oh, go ahead and take it out."

The elderly woman spun around to her daughter and snapped, "Mind your own business!"

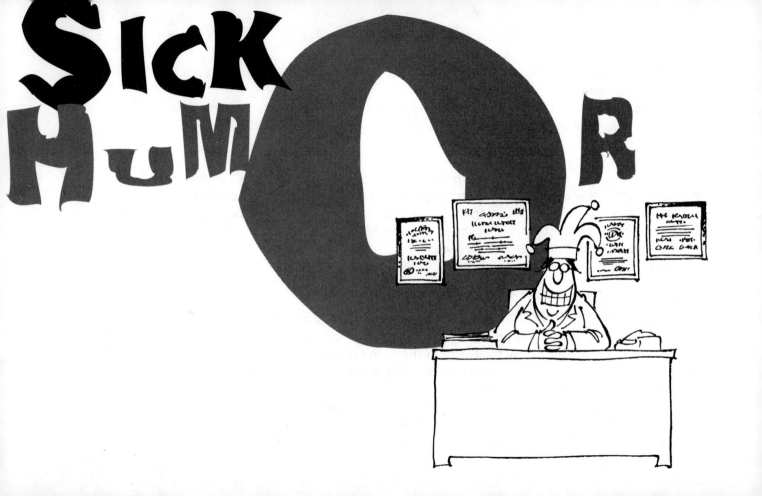

The Doctor's Office

What a Bedside Manner

Dr. J. Banks Hankins of Lexington, North Carolina, had just completed a pelvic exam of a young woman on whom he had recently done a hysterectomy for carcinoma of the cervix.

Since she was the quiet type, the doctor assumed she was very shy.

As he removed his glove following the pelvic exam, Dr. Hankins told his patient, "Well, I don't see anything there to get excited about."

She looked at him square in the eyes and said in a mock hurt voice, "Why, Doctor, that's the most unflattering thing anyone ever said to me!"

Never go to a doctor whose plants have died.

— Erma Bombeck, *columnist*

The Wrong End

It was one of those days when Dr. William A. Calderwood of Sun City, Arizona, didn't have time to relax for a moment. All the examining rooms were full, and so was the waiting room. Naturally, the phone was ringing constantly.

The harried doctor had a patient all ready for her pap smear and pelvic exam. At the propitious moment of insertion of the speculum, he momentarily lost his train of thought and said, "Say 'Aah.'"

Not believing her ears, the patient replied, "What did you say?"

Recalled Dr. Calderwood years later, "There's no graceful way out of that situation."

Who's the Doctor Here?

The nurse for gynecologist Jon S. Nielson of Minneapolis asks return patients to partially disrobe after they enter the examination room and wait for the doctor.

But it's his standard practice that a first-time patient remain fully clothed in the exam room while she waits for him. When he meets her for the first time, he introduces himself and takes her history. Then he stands up and says, "I'll leave the room, you get undressed, and I'll be back in a couple of minutes."

One busy day, following an exhausting all-night obstetrical vigil, Dr. Nielson got his words mixed up during his first meeting with a new patient. He told the young woman sitting in front of him, "I'll leave and get undressed and be back in a couple of minutes."

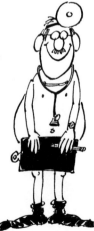

What a Card!

A young and very attractive woman who worked for American Express went to see Dr. Philip D. Windrow.

After completing a pelvic exam on her, the doctor fitted the patient with a diaphragm that she had requested. When he explained its use, she asked him if he had any further instructions.

Dr. Windrow couldn't resist. His words of advice to the diaphragm-wearing American Express employee: "Don't leave home without it!"

Over His Head—Both Times

As an intern, Dr. Michael A. Stillman of Mount Kisco, New York, was assigned to a clinic to see patients who didn't have a private physician.

One day, he was examining a man and found a heart condition that the intern felt was beyond his expertise. Dr. Stillman told his patient that he didn't feel qualified to diagnose the problem and referred the patient to the cardiology clinic. The intern even called and made an appointment for the patient for a couple of weeks later.

A week or so later, Dr. Stillman completed his rotation in internal medicine and was transferred to cardiology. And who became his first heart patient? Much to the patient's chagrin and to the intern's embarrassment, it was the very same man that Dr. Stillman had sent to the cardiology clinic!

Doctor, Are You Okay?

Dr. Wiley K. Livingston Jr. of Bessemer, Alabama, frequently admits patients of dubious mental status whom he subjects to the time-honored question sequence of date, location, and identity of the president of the United States.

One evening in 1991, he admitted an elderly woman through the emergency room. Because she was new to him and the doctor was uncertain of her orientation, he quickly ran her through the test.

"Mrs. Smith," he asked, "do you know where we are?" She correctly identified the hospital and the city.

"Well, then, perhaps you can tell me the date," said the doctor. Once again, her answer was correct.

"Very good," Dr. Livingston. "Now one more question. Who is the president of the United States?"

"George Bush," she replied.

Satisfied that all was well, Dr. Livingston started to leave when Mrs. Smith called him back. "Doctor," she said a little concerned, "have you figured out where *you* are? You seem awfully confused."

A male gynecologist is like an auto mechanic who has never owned a car.
— Carrie Snow, *comedienne*

Limited Practice

A patient, alarmed by her husband's breaking of furniture and other violent behavior, persuaded Dr. Raymond C. Maronpot of Bernardsville, New Jersey, to come see him at their home.

The patient's barely repressed hostility made the doctor suspect advanced paranoia. Dr. Maronpot finally convinced him to go for a psychiatric consultation with another doctor.

The day after the patient's appointment, the consulting psychiatrist phoned Dr. Maronpot. "Ray," he said, "never send anyone like him again. This guy is crazy."

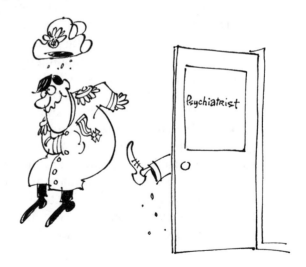

The Spirit of Christmas

One snowy, cold Christmas Eve after the kids were in bed, Dr. Arnold R. Murray of Calgary, Alberta, helped his wife June finish wrapping the gifts. The couple relaxed in front of the fireplace and listened to carols on the stereo.

Dr. Murray soon became aware of a car horn honking incessantly. Looking up through the window, he told June, "Some jackass has spun around on the corner and sunk the back end of his car in a snowbank. It must be four feet into the snow. Probably drunk. Probably wants me to come and dig him out. Forget it, chum! Dig yourself out."

The doctor turned his attention back to the Christmas carols when he noticed that the honking had stopped. Once again, he peered out the window.

"He's drunk, June. He's standing on the side of the motor steadying himself with one hand on the hood and using an axe with the other. He must be loaded. Well, he's on his way and when he gets to the door we can call a cab for him."

Then Dr. Murray stood back and admired the mound of presents that surrounded the Christmas tree. The couple reflected on how fortunate they were to have six children and the means to provide for them. By now it was 2 A.M. After turning off the lights and heading for bed, Dr. Murray suddenly remembered the drunk in the street. The man had yet to knock on the door.

Dr. Murray went to the window and saw the man in the middle of the road, belly down, doing a breast stroke as if he was trying to swim across the icy, snowy street. Worried that the man could be run over or freeze to death, Dr. Murray rushed outside to help.

When the doctor reached him, the man gasped, "I thought you'd never come. And when you turned out the lights, I almost died. I spun my car around on the ice and when it hit the snow-bank, I broke my leg. And I only had two small drinks. Thank God you came!"

Dr. Murray and his wife wrapped the man in blankets, carefully placed him on a toboggan, loaded him into the family station wagon, and rushed him to the hospital. Within an hour, Dr. Murray had the fractured leg put in a cast.

Years later, Dr. Murray recalled, "As I drove home, I made an effort to think about the spirit of Christmas and how I'd almost lost it."

It's a good idea to "shop around" before you settle on a doctor. Ask about the condition of his Mercedes. Ask about the competence of his mechanic. Don't be shy! After all, you're paying for it.

— Dave Barry, *humorist*

The Sexpert

A colleague of Dr. Marion Rogers of Vancouver, British Columbia, once was asked by his wife's luncheon group to be their guest speaker.

When he told his wife that he decided to talk about waterskiing, she scoffed and said that he didn't know the first thing about the sport. On the day of his speech, his wife was sitting in the audience. When he was introduced, she muttered to friends at her table that she didn't intend to sit there and listen to her husband make a fool of himself. She got up and went into the lobby.

As the doctor took the podium, he looked around and noticed an obviously bright, young group of women. He felt a sudden wave of insecurity, despite his research into waterskiing. So he decided at the last moment to talk about something he really understood—sex.

The doctor gave an excellent presentation, drawing ad lib from his experiences in gynecological practice. When the luncheon was over, several women met his wife in the lobby and told her how great he was as a speaker and how well he had covered the subject.

She snorted in disbelief. And what she said next had the women stunned in similar disbelief. "For heaven's sake," she said. "He's only done it twice—and he fell off both times."

It's Only Skin Deep

When Dr. Patricia Mark of Lantzville, British Columbia, first went into general practice years ago, a grubby, incredibly hairy young man came in for an examination.

He told her that he had some concerns "down there." But he wouldn't elaborate. Further questions from Dr. Mark produced no other details. It was clear that, having received his relevant history, she needed to inspect "down there." Conjuring up all sorts of nameless horrors that might exist, the physician didn't really want to put her fingers "down there."

Suddenly, Dr. Mark came up with a creative solution. "What you need," she said, "is a specialist." She then hurried to the front desk, thrust the patient's chart into the hands of the startled receptionist, and told her to get an urgent appointment with the local urologist.

Feeling remarkably pleased with the way she handled the situation, Dr. Mark didn't give the matter another thought until a few weeks later, when she received a letter from the urologist.

"Thank you for sending Mr. ____ along, and for your helpful information," said the letter. "On examination, I find that he has a couple of warts on his lower abdomen and have taken the liberty of sending him along to the dermatologist."

For Dr. Mark, it was most embarrassing. And the urologist has never let her forget it either.

No Way Out

Dr. A.K. Bowles of Kanata, Ontario, referred a fifteen-year-old girl to a plastic surgeon for the removal of a small mole on her cheek.

Accompanied by her mother, the patient arrived in her school uniform—white blouse, knee-length pleated plaid skirt with matching tie and kneesocks—and perched on the examining table. Her mother sat in a nearby chair.

After looking at the mole, Dr. Bowles answered the mother's questions and concerns. In great detail, he explained the need for stitches, the size and shape of the scar, and the expected amount of blood loss. At that point, the girl, who had remained sitting on the examining table, turned pale and fainted. She fell backward into a recessed window and landed upside down in a glass alcove that projected out from the room of the high-rise building.

Her mother panicked and began screaming, spurring the doctor to leap onto the examining table. He placed the girl's knees around his waist, grasped her thighs firmly and tried to yank up his unconsciousness patient. But he failed and she remained upside down. However, enough blood had rushed to her head that she began recovering from her fainting spell.

Imagine the poor girl's shock when she found herself in a bizarre predicament: stuck upside down, looking over a parking lot seven stories below, her skirt up to her chin, her mother screaming hysterically in the background, and her doctor forcefully pulling on her separated thighs. Not surprisingly, the girl began to scream and struggle violently.

Hearing the commotion, the doctor's nurse ran into the room. There was the mother jumping up and down, shrieking, and the doctor kneeling on the examining table straddled by two furiously kicking legs. Realizing it wasn't what it appeared, the nurse leaped onto the table and helped the doctor extricate the patient.

But there was no way the patient, mother, or doctor could extricate themselves from the embarrassment.

A Mountain of Trouble

Years ago, an intern was in the operating room with a resident gynecologist who was doing a D&C on an extremely obese patient.

In those days, the operating table could easily be moved around. On this particular morning, the table was not centered properly under the light. The resident asked that the table be shoved a little closer to the middle of the room. The patient weighed so much, however, that the surgical team could not move the table. So the gynecologist had to move his wheeled stool to the patient.

The intern couldn't help himself. He blurted out, "This is really a case of when the mountain won't go to Mohammed, Mohammed must go to the mountain."

* * *

A hospital's chief of staff told two surgery residents that they would have to perform an appendectomy on a patient by themselves.

The patient turned out to be an extremely obese woman whose abdomen hung over both sides of the surgical table. The two young doctors confidently made the incision over the area where they thought the appendix would be. But as they cut deeper and deep through the fat, they failed to reach any internal organs.

They started to get concerned—especially when they cut deeper and found something green. A moment later, they realized what it was—the sterile green sheet under the patient! The doctors had cut all the way through the patient and totally missed her organs. They sewed up the original incision—front and back—and moved several inches to the right. They finally came upon the appendix and removed it without further incident.

The patient made a fine recovery—and never asked why she had an extra scar on both her abdomen and her back.

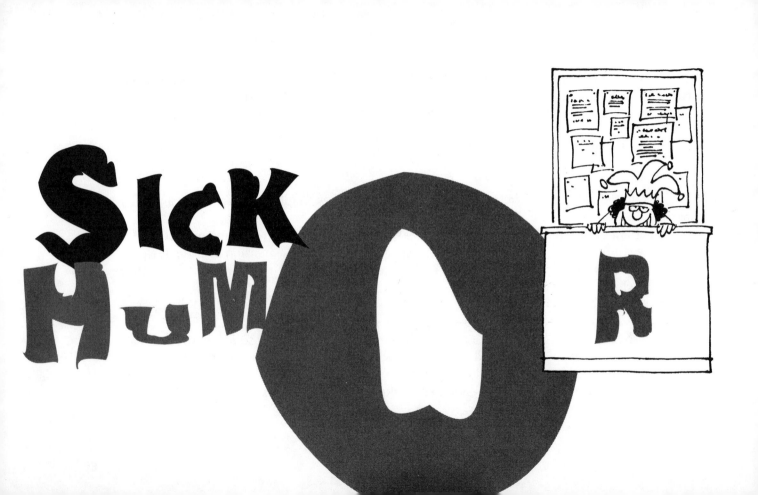

The Nurses' Station

A Heartfelt Thanks but No Thanks

Several times over a two-week period a patient on the telemetry unit needed his heart shocked or chest thumped. Since there was no physician present at these times, the nurses did the procedures without giving sedation. Consequently, the patient would usually let out a loud yell.

Fred, a big strong charge nurse, had thumped and shocked the patient the most. The patient complained he didn't know which was worse—the thumping or the shocking.

One night while working as the charge nurse, Thomas Steeves answered a code. It was the same patient. Noticing the unit's defibrillator was dead, Steeves asked Fred to bring another cart. When the patient saw Fred enter the room, he gave himself a thump on the chest—and got his heart back into a normal rhythm.

Explaining his actions, the patient pointed to Fred and said, "I just didn't want him hitting me again."

Measuring Up to the Task

Certain staff members at a community hospital where Mildred Thompson worked were assigned numbers for paging purposes.

According to Mildred, a young, slender nurse, who transferred to a job requiring such a code, was instructed to select one for herself.

"There's a number I've always wanted to be," she said enthusiastically.

Imagine everyone's amusement when the slight-of-build nurse was paged over the intercom: "38D, please . . . 38D."

Number, Please

Hospital codes over the intercom are designed so they alert the staff without alarming the patients.

But sometimes those codes can be confusing, as it was for one nurse at a hospital in Tempe, Arizona.

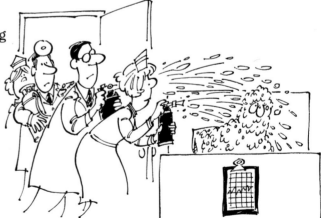

Hospitals have codes to describe events that you don't want to broadcast to everyone in English. For example, you might hear "Code 1,000, Room 202." That's better than hearing, "The patient in 202 has just died."

A new nurse had trouble remembering what each code meant and often got the codes mixed up. One day, while she was on duty, a patient's heart stopped. The nurse picked up the phone and shouted, "Code 5,000, Room 312." The operator broadcast the information, and moments later, about forty people carrying fire extinguishers ran to the room of the coded patient. Only then did the nurse realize she had given the code for fire.

A month later, the hospital changed the codes to the less confusing "Code Blue" and "Code Red."

Reality Check

Betty Cissna of Medford, Oregon, was a staff nurse on a surgical floor that was often quite busy.

One day, the floor was bustling more than usual. So many people were scheduled for surgery in the morning that by the afternoon the nurses were tied up returning postoperative patients to their rooms. The nurses didn't have time to respond to other patients' every whim.

At 2 P.M., the patient intercom buzzed at the nurse's desk. Loud and clear, the staff heard an annoyed patient declare, "*General Hospital* is on TV. I want all of you to come to my room and see how a *real* hospital is run!"

Missing the Mark

Nursing instructor Linda Rooda, Ph.D. and RN, was watching a student try to give her first injection to a patient.

Hoping to calm the nervous student, Linda held the subcutaneous tissue so the student could concentrate on getting the medication directly into the muscle. Linda then watched in horror as the student swiftly plunged the needle slightly off-target through the outstretched webbing between Linda's thumb and forefinger and into the patient. The student then depressed the plunger and removed the needle.

When they left the patient, Linda nursed her sore hand and waited for an apology. She was surprised to discover that the student had failed to notice that needle had joined the instructor to the patient. Trying to remain cool, Linda explained what had taken place. The student was so shocked and embarrassed that she hid in the employee bathroom for the rest of the afternoon.

* * *

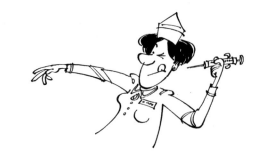

On a student's first day of taking vital signs, she ran up to Linda and declared that her patient didn't have a pulse.

Linda raced into the room and found an elderly woman reading the *Wall Street Journal*. Assuring the student that the patient had a pulse, Linda asked the student to take the pulse again.

The student placed the bell of the stethoscope in the lower left quadrant of the patient's abdominal area. Asked why she chose that site for finding the pulse, the student replied, "Mrs. Rooda, you said to place the bell of the stethoscope approximately one inch below the nipple line."

"Yes, that's true," said Linda, realizing that as an instructor she had neglected to address situations where the breasts of elderly women hang below their navels. Linda then made a mental note: *Never underestimate the ability of a beginning student to take me literally.*

It's a lot harder to keep people well than it is to just get them over a sickness.

— DeForest Clinton Jarvis, *contemporary writer*

Perhaps You're a Little Too Focused

Soon after nursing student Lisa Pitler learned the proper technique for a bed bath, she was assigned to her first nursing home patient. The elderly man was sleeping and badly in need of a bath.

Lisa, now a registered nurse, cautiously wrapped the washcloth, as instructed, to avoid dripping water on the patient. With total concentration, she began to bathe him.

Lisa was doing his feet when her instructor entered the room and asked, "How's the bath going?"

"It's going just fine," Lisa replied.

"Has the patient moved or made any noise during the procedure?"

"No," said Lisa. "He's been quiet and seems to be enjoying the bath."

The instructor took Lisa out into the hall and then told her, "The patient you were bathing expired several hours ago."

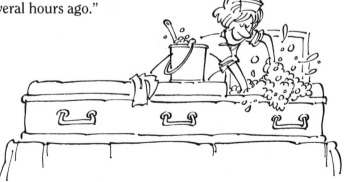

Letting it All Hang Out

Student nurse Julie Heaton-Hill was told to bathe a frail eighty-year-old man in a special chair which had a hole in the bottom for water to drain.

Julie loaded him up, using good body mechanics. She covered him with warm blankets, wrapped his feet, and took all the shower things she needed for a single trip down the hall to the shower area.

Julie was feeling quite proud of herself until her instructor stopped her and pulled her back a few steps. Pointing to the patient, the instructor asked Julie, "What's wrong with this picture?"

Julie thought a moment. *What could possibly be the problem? Blankets? Check. Shower supplies? Check. Feet covered? Check. Uh-oh . . . What is that dangling out from the shower chair hole? Come to think of it, he had mentioned feeling a draft.*

Clowning Around

In the hospital where registered nurse Kalynn Pressly worked, one of the chaplains was a jolly Episcopal priest with a ruddy complexion and bright red curly hair. He was somewhat unconventional in his manner and attire, but his ministry was appreciated by both patients and staff.

One morning he entered the ICU wearing hiking boots, mustard colored pants, and a pale orange shirt with a clerical collar. He came into the room of a slightly confused patient whose vital signs were being checked by Kalynn. The priest talked with them for a few minutes.

After the priest left the room, the patient told Kalynn, "I think it's really nice of the hospital to hire clowns to entertain the patients."

After two days in the hospital, I took a turn for the nurse.

— W. C. Fields, *comedian*

Dead to the World

Serena Miller worked the midnight shift as an emergency room clerk in the Vanderbilt University Medical Center in Nashville.

One night, around 3 A.M., she saw several obnoxious students walk in to watch the doctors and nurses in action. After trying unsuccessfully to get the students to leave, Serena dialed what she thought was the campus police.

When a sleepy male voice answered, Serena asked, "Would you come and pick up several people who are just lying around, cluttering up the emergency room?"

"How many are there?" he asked in a strained voice.

Puzzled by the question, Serena told him, "We hadn't bothered to count them."

After a long pause, the man said, "Lady, I sure hope you've got the wrong number. This is the Woodlawn Funeral Home."

Bump and Run

As acting coroner, Dr. Francis N. Taylor of Petersburg, Virginia, came to the hospital late one night to check on the victim of a fatal accident.

An orderly accompanied him down the dimly lit hall in the basement that led to the morgue. Aware that the pathologist sometimes worked behind a locked door, Dr. Taylor knocked three times.

Seeing this, the spooked orderly declared, "If anyone answers, I'm leaving!"

Getting the Name Straight

Dr. John H. Hirsh of Fort Lauderdale reported that a hostile young lady, apparently high on drugs, went to the emergency room desk, complaining of pain in her arm.

The clerk asked for her name. Rather than give it, the patient responded with a common vulgarism.

The unflappable clerk then asked, "Do you spell that with an 'F' or 'Ph'?"

Creative Triage

It was a busy night in the emergency room at Toronto's East General Hospital.

A.C. Stone of Windsor, Ontario, reported that patients waiting to be treated filled the waiting room. Suddenly a man cradling a possible broken finger bulled his way to the receptionist's desk and demanded to be X-rayed immediately.

The young lady explained to him that some of the others had been waiting for more than an hour and so he would have to wait his turn. But he refused to listen and became belligerent. "I don't care about the others!" he stormed. "I've got things to do. I can't be sitting around here all night. I want this finger X-rayed right now!"

Again, the receptionist tried to explain that his injury didn't warrant moving him to the front of the line. The man still demanded immediate attention. As he became more and more abusive, she stood up, walked around the counter, took him by the arm, and marched him to the center of the waiting room.

As the other patients looked up, the receptionist said, "Excuse me, ladies and gentlemen. Can I have your attention for a moment? This gentleman is a very busy person and feels that qualifies him to be treated ahead of the rest of you. How do you feel about that?"

Given the response from those who had been patiently waiting their turns, the complainer suddenly decided that his finger didn't need to be X-rayed after all.

A Disturbing Diagnosis

An urgent care receptionist for Dr. Edward A. Ortiz, then of Lakeland, Florida, followed proper procedure by recording a patient's chief complaint on a slip of paper, which was in the patient's own words. The receptionist then passed the information to a nurse for an assessment.

When she brought the nurse the slip of paper, the receptionist had a perplexed look on her face.

"What's wrong?" asked the nurse.

"This lady's ear and the side of her face are swollen and red," the receptionist replied. "She says she's had it before and that it's called ear syphilis.

"I want to know one thing," said the receptionist, who wasn't aware that the correct term for this condition is erysipelas. "Just how do you get this?"

A Heavy Caseload

When Dr. Ralph G. Bennett of Hayward, California, ran out of antifungal powder in his dermatology office, he learned that his regular supplier was back-ordered.

Dr. Bennett wanted some immediately, so he sent one of his staffers to buy all she could find at a nearby drugstore. As she deposited all thirteen containers on the checkout counter, the clerk did a double-take and exclaimed, "Gosh, lady, you must have some problem!"

Safety First

Dr. Jose J. Llinas of Gainesville, Florida, reported that when the season opened for hunters to infiltrate the dense woods surrounding his hospital, this warning appeared on the employees' bulletin board:

PLEASE REMAIN ON THE HOSPITAL GROUNDS AND STAY OUT OF THE WOODS WHERE YOU MIGHT BE MISTAKEN FOR A DEER AND SHOT. THAT WOULD GENERATE A LOT OF EXTRA PAPERWORK AND ADVERSELY AFFECT THE CURRENT STAFFING PATTERN.

Inflation Is Part of Life

One day at lunch in the Department of Health and Human Services cafeteria, a group of attorneys for the federal Health Care Financing Administration was discussing the case of a transsexual.

The attorney handling the case said the transsexual was seeking to have Medicare pay for the reconstructive surgery involved in the transition from female to male. When the attorney described the inflatable device that was implanted in the newly-constructed penis, there were a few guffaws.

Recalled one of the members of the luncheon group that day, "Apparently we had grown just a bit louder in our now somewhat risqué discussion. Embarrassingly, we drew the attention of the secretary of Human Services herself, then the Honorable Margaret Heckler, who came along and joined us at the table, asking what we were finding so humorous.

"After a couple of moments of awkward silence, the attorney who had been telling us of the penile implant and inflation techniques began to somewhat hesitatingly relate what we had been discussing. He described how the penile implant was inflated by hand.

"To my eternal memory, the secretary hardly missed a beat when she commented, 'Isn't that the way it is usually done?'"

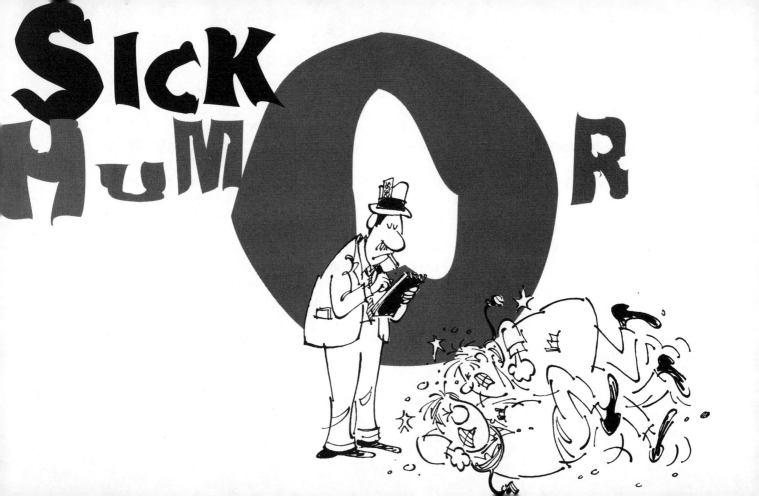

The Rounds
(of Weird Medical News)

Surgeons Brawl as Patient Snoozes

While a patient was out cold on the operating table, two doctors were duking it out on the operating room floor.

The medical mayhem erupted on October 24, 1991, at the Medical Center of Central Massachusetts in Worcester. According to a subsequent medical board hearing, here is what happened:

Surgeon Dr. Mohan Korgaonkar, forty-nine, was about to begin surgery on an elderly woman when he and anesthesiologist Dr. Kwok Wei Chan, forty-three, started to argue. Dr. Chan swore at Dr. Korgaonkar, who responded by throwing a cotton-tipped prep stick at the anesthesiologist. The two raised their fists at each other and engaged in a scuffle that sent both to the floor.

While they were battling on the floor, a shocked nurse had the presence of mind to monitor the sleeping patient. When the doctors finally came to their senses and quit fighting, they resumed the operation, which was completed a half hour later without incident. The patient didn't find out about the operating room altercation until after her recovery.

When the hospital learned of the brawl, it placed the doctors on five years' probation.

So who won the fight? Looking into the matter two years later, the state Board of Registration in Medicine came up with a split decision. It fined the pugilistic physicians $10,000 each and ordered them to undergo joint psychotherapy.

Doctor Saves Own Life by Jolting Himself

A doctor whose heart was beating wildly survived by zapping himself with two high-powered electrical jolts from his office defibrillator.

In 1995, Dr. Jean Cukier, a forty-year-old plastic surgeon from Houston, received a nasty shock when he pulled a burning lamp cord from an outlet in his office. The shock sent his heart racing at 160 beats per minute and left him extremely dizzy.

Fearing that he faced serious heart problems, Dr. Cukier yelled for his assistant and then dragged himself to his office operating room. With his assistant's help, the doctor smeared himself with conductor jelly, lay on the operating table, and placed the defibrillator paddles on his chest.

The defibrillator uses a powerful burst of electricity to restore the heart to a normal beat after cardiac arrest or other rhythm abnormalities. The machine is hardly designed for self-use.

But Dr. Cukier felt he had no choice. He was about to lose consciousness when he turned on the juice. The first jolt threw him off the table, but failed to correct his rapid heartbeat. Incredibly, the determined physician managed to climb back onto the operating table and tried defibbing himself again. Fortunately, this time, it worked.

Dr. Cukier later told the press that his self-diagnosis was atrial fibrillation, which he called a "potentially life-threatening" condition that might not have responded well to medication.

"Treating it conservatively was taking a chance because your heart can clot when it's irregular," he said. "Then the clots shoot up into your brain."

Dr. Amin Karim of Baylor College of Medicine in Houston eventually treated Dr. Cukier, whose amazing self-rescue was described in the *New England Journal of Medicine.*

Dr. Karim said that Dr.Cukier probably would have been better off dialing 911 for an ambulance.

"It was very daring," said Dr. Karim. "What if he had passed out? He could have put himself into a more dangerous rhythm. If that happened, it would have meant cardiac arrest. It ended up saving his life, but it could have gone the other way.

"Don't try this at home."

Physician Loses His Heads

Dr. William Portney lost his heads. That's right, heads.

According to the Associated Press, Dr. Portney, of New York, was transporting a box of human heads in 1991 for use in a dissection class. Thinking they wouldn't fit in a laboratory refrigerator, he left them in his car overnight in Manhattan's East Village.

That night, thieves broke into his trunk. They snatched the box and took off. But apparently when they opened the box up and saw the gruesome contents, they freaked out. They dropped the box in a gutter and fled.

A curious cab driver, Gheorghe Casas, saw them dump the box and went to investigate. When he discovered the heads, he stashed them in his trunk and called police.

The heads were returned to Dr. Portney once he proved legal ownership.

Doctor Quits for Life as Truck Driver

Overworked and stressed out, Dr. Deborah Janicki wrote herself a prescription in 1992—she quit her practice to become a truck driver.

Deborah was putting in sixteen- to twenty-hour days as the only doctor in Marengo, Iowa, when she got fed up with medicine. "I was being worked to death," she told reporters. "I was holding down my practice single-handedly, plus covering the emergency room at Marengo Memorial Hospital.

"I never got enough sleep. My blood pressure soared and I had stomach problems. Besides that, I was short and snappy with people. Finally, one day I said to myself, 'Take a look at your life.'"

So at the age of forty-one, with no husband or children to worry about, Deborah quit her $85,000-a-year practice and enrolled in a truck driving school. Months later, she began driving an eighteen-wheeler, hauling a fifty-three-foot trailer five thousand miles a week. Said Deborah at the time, "It's not an easy job. But compared to what I was doing, it's heaven."

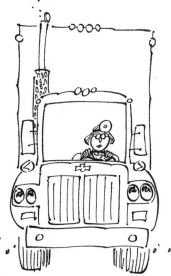

America's Funniest Dentist

Dr. Steven Stutsman of Dallas was named America's Funniest Dentist in 1992 with good reason. He makes his patients laugh—without using gas.

In fact, he relies on humor to ease anxious patients and to establish rapport.

Many times, after delivering the local anesthetic, Dr. Stutsman will pat the patient on the shoulder and leave the room, mumbling, "I'll be right back. I need to go back to my office for a second to read up on how to do this."

After the patient takes a few seconds deciding whether or not to panic, the dental assistant will break up laughing—and the patient lets out a sigh of relief.

* * *

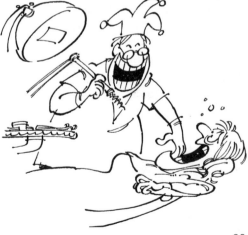

Sometimes a patient shows up and tells Dr. Stutsman, "I'm sorry, Doctor, but I've been so busy running around that I didn't get a chance to brush my teeth." When he hears that excuse, the dentist replies sympathetically, "I know how it is. I've been so busy I haven't had a chance to wash my hands."

* * *

Patients often ask Dr. Stutsman if he uses nitrous oxide during dental procedures. "I most certainly do," he answers. "Eventually, I'm going to let patients start using it too."

Docs Aren't What They're Quacked Up to Be

Not all doctors are who they say they are.

A new general practitioner at a Leningrad clinic quickly became the patients' favorite doctor in 1990. They liked him because he usually prescribed tea, honey, and long sick leaves.

But his own popularity landed him in jail—because he was a fraud.

According to the Communist Party newspaper *Pravda,* Fyodor Kuznetsov, thirty, worked as a piano tuner, salesman, and cloakroom attendant. But then he forged documents to get a job as a physician in a clinic.

His treatment, which included "very generous" sick leaves, became so popular, said the newspaper, that his patients requested his picture be hung at the Health Ministry. Several extremely pleased patients even wrote to *Pravda* praising his work.

As a result of the doctor's popularity, an author was interested in writing his biography, even though Kuznetsov had been at the clinic for only four months. When the author started researching the doctor's life, it became obvious that Kuznetsov was a fake.

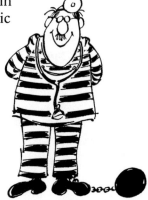

Authorities gave him a dose of harsh reality—a jail cell for pretending to be a doctor.

* * *

Decked out in a white gown, blue surgical cap, and a stethoscope, Dr. Navarro seemed what he appeared to be—a physician who practiced at two hospitals in San Bernardino County, California.

But he was really David Aaron Green—a state prison parolee who had been previously convicted of practicing medicine without a license.

His downfall came in 1993 when he dated a nurse. As luck would have it, on their first date they came upon a traffic accident. The nurse noted Green inappropriately put first-aid cream on a child's serious head injury. (Fortunately, the child was not harmed by the faulty treatment.)

The nurse became even more suspicious when she tried to reach him the next day. Referring to the business card he had given her, the nurse called his office and asked for Dr. Corazon Navarro.

"She's not in," said a member of Dr. Navarro's staff.

When the nurse learned that the real Dr. Navarro was a woman, she immediately contacted authorities in Sacramento. Police arrested Green on suspicion of impersonating a doctor. They picked him up at the airport, where he was wearing a stethoscope around his neck.

* * *

A daring imposter treated dozens of people at four different Cincinnati hospitals for at least three years before he was caught.

Oddly enough, he never took a dime from his patients for his services.

The saga of Thomas West began in 1983 when the former bank employee started a company to help doctors manage their offices. To learn more about the profession, he began sneaking into lectures at the University of Cincinnati College of Medicine in 1986. He even joined the daily hospital rounds wearing a lab coat and stethoscope and staff doctors assumed he was a medical student.

In 1988, West began introducing himself to potential clients for his management business as "Dr. West" and started treating friends and acquaintances for free. He simply walked into emergency rooms, pretending to be a physician. He used fake ID cards and stole prescription pads. According to authorities, West performed minor surgery, prescribed medication, conducted Pap smears, and even delivered a baby.

In 1991, a patient learned from West's landlord that his "doctor" was about to be evicted for not paying his rent. Suspicious, the patient called police, who conducted an investigation that revealed West was a phony.

West was sentenced to three years in prison for practicing medicine without a license. After serving eighteen months, he came out, but was sent back to prison after he tried to start a new career—impersonating a lawyer!

College Student Cuts Out Own Tonsils

In 1992, Poppy Faldmo, a communications major at Salt Lake Community College in Utah, was fed up by the recurring strep throats and abscesses she had suffered since childhood. Neither she nor her family could afford health insurance for her and she didn't have the $1,500 needed to pay for a tonsillectomy. So she took matters into her own hands—and throat.

Poppy used a trial and error method to remove her tonsils a bit at a time over several weeks. Before the first operation, Poppy shined a flashlight down her throat and examined her tonsils while looking at her makeup mirror. They were badly inflamed. "I was scared and trembling," she recalled. "But I told myself, 'Be careful, you can do it.'"

According to the *National Enquirer,* the twenty-one-year-old student snipped away her tonsils using cuticle scissors, an Exacto knife, and tweezers. Tooth-numbing medication served as a local anesthetic. To stop the bleeding, she cauterized the incisions by scorching them with a red-hot metal rod and an electric wood-engraving tool.

"I operated on myself about twenty times and never missed school," she said, adding, "I haven't had a problem since I finished."

At the *Enquirer*'s expense, Poppy was examined by Dr. Keith Finlayson, an ear, nose, and throat specialist in Salt Lake City. The doctor noted there was still some tonsil tissue Poppy had failed to remove. Added the doctor, "I've never seen anyone do anything like this."

The Hospital from Hell

What was supposed to be a vacation in paradise for Hollywood actor Gary Griffith turned into a nightmare in the hospital from hell.

During a 1992 vacation on the tiny Fiji island of Nananu-i-Ra, Gary was wading in the ocean when he was stung on his left foot by a poisonous stonefish. Burning with fever and pain, Gary was rushed by the hotel staff to a larger Fiji island where he was admitted to the hospital.

"But my frightening ordeal was just beginning," he told reporters later. "This so-called hospital was more like a butcher shop. The doctors and nurses were amateurs and medication was a joke.

"A nurse would simply hand me a tray of pills and tell me to take what I needed because she wasn't sure when she'd be back. The staff even offered me marijuana cigarettes!"

Gary's leg had swelled up so badly that the doctors considered amputating it. He begged them to call an American doctor, but they said the phones didn't work.

"Doctors then decided to do exploratory surgery and I remember being wheeled into a filthy operating room," Gary recalled. "The next thing I knew it was three days later. A nurse said I'd been given too much anesthesia. My heart had stopped on the table and I'd almost died."

Gary was just as shocked when he discovered that the surgeons had cut a large chunk out of his foot and hadn't even stitched or bandaged the gaping wound. "Suddenly the thought struck me, 'I'm going to die if I don't get home.'"

The next day, Gary stole a cleaning lady's broom for a crutch and hobbled over to a food cart. Then he tried to roll himself out of the hospital. He barely made it past the lobby. Hospital officials, worried about getting paid, summoned Fijian soldiers who brought Gary back to his room.

After two weeks of agony, Gary sneaked out of the hospital with the help of a friendly nurse and her doctor husband. Gary caught a flight to Honolulu where, with a 105-degree fever, he was admitted to Queen's Medical Center. He was released five weeks later. Upon his return to Los Angeles, Gary underwent an operation to remove a piece of the stonefish's stinger that was still embedded in a bone in his foot.

Gary was finally able to walk normally again three months after he fled the hospital from hell.

Woman Undergoes Plastic Surgery Eighteen Times for the Right Look

Cindy Jackson spent $55,000 on eighteen operations in four years just to get the right look.

"You can't buy love, but you can buy lovely," she told reporters in London in 1992. "I used my money to make my childhood dream come true.

"People stop me on the street and tell me I look just like Barbie with my turned-up nose and pouted lips. That makes me feel great."

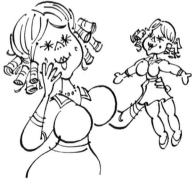

Cindy, who was born and raised on a farm in Ohio, said she never felt pretty growing up or as an adult—until she underwent her surgical transformation in London. "I thought I was ugly," she admitted. "My nose was too big, my lips too thin, my eyes too small and hooded. I had a mean-looking mouth and a double chin. My chest was flat and I had a bulging stomach. I had saddlebags on my hips and thighs and even my knees were fat.

"I wasn't pretty or sensuous. Then my father died and left me some money—and with that and my savings, I started transforming myself into my dream girl."

Cindy had her eyes lifted and followed that with liposuction, upper and lower face-lifts, chemical peels, tummy tucks, breast implants, two nose jobs, and other cosmetic surgery. She had some procedures more than once.

"I'm proud of myself," she said. "I was a hick from the sticks. But I had a dream and made it come true."

Man . . . Hic . . . Has Suffered . . . Hic . . . since 1960

Back in 1960, John Crosland started hiccuping for no apparent reason. He assumed they would go away. They didn't. In fact, they've been with him ever since.

"I've tried every remedy imaginable," said the fifty-eight-year-old victim from Laurinburg, North Carolina. "I've drunk gallons of water, breathed into paper bags, held my breath. I even stood on my head.

"Everyone and his brother have suggested a cure—and I've tried most of them. I've also taken a number of prescription medications over the years. But nothing works."

The hiccups are at their worst for Crosland when he gets up in the morning. They usually come every two seconds during the first ten minutes that he's awake. Then they taper off to about one every minute or so. The only time he doesn't hiccup is when he sleeps.

By hiccuping virtually every minute of his waking hours since 1960, it's estimated that Crosland had hiccuped nearly twelve million times by 1995.

Nevertheless, Crosland, the married father of six children, has been in pretty good health and learned to live with his condition. In fact, hiccups are such a part of his life that he's not sure he wants them to stop. "If they did," he said, "I'd wonder what was wrong."

Life Was the Pits

When Francis Reichert was eight years old, he liked showing off to the other kids in the neighborhood by stuffing cherry pits up each nostril. He'd then blow the pits out.

But one day, he had to sniff—and one of the cherry pits got wedged in his right nostril. Try as he might, he couldn't get that nasty pit out of his nose. It was really starting to bug him. Finally, he had to confess.

"I told my mother, and got in trouble," recalled Francis, of Stuart, Florida. "Three weeks later, I was still complaining" that the cherry pit was lodged in his nose. "My mother took me to the doctor, but he didn't find anything."

So Francis learned to live with the slight discomfort in his right nostril.

But then, fifty years after the cherry pit incident, Francis went to Dr. Richard Perrotta, an ear, nose, and throat specialist in Stuart. "He poked and prodded and suddenly the pit dropped in my mouth," Francis recalled.

After finding the pit tucked far up the patient's nose, Dr. Perrotta was stunned to learn how long it had been up there. He told the *Palm Beach Post* he may report the case to medical journals because he believes the centimeter-long calcified pit may be the oldest object discovered in anyone's nose.

Instead of pits, Francis now had to contend with ribs—especially from his coworkers at the Martin County Property Appraiser's Office. Laughed Francis, "They started saying I had pits for brains."

Physician Collars Mysterious Malady

While driving on the freeway in Los Angeles, John J. Fried looked over his left shoulder when suddenly he began to black out.

He turned his head to the right and quickly regained consciousness, although his heart was pounding furiously. Knowing that something was terribly wrong, he underwent a variety of tests and was even outfitted with a portable heart monitor. Ten days later, the results came back: His heart was in great shape.

But then one day, while walking to lunch, he turned and looked down at something on the sidewalk. Once again, he nearly passed out. Worried that he might have a brain tumor or was afflicted with tiny strokes or seizures, John described the incidents to a doctor friend.

The physician's prescription: Buy shirts with bigger collar sizes. Apparently, when John turned his head on the freeway and when he was walking, his shirt collar dug into his neck and stimulated the vagus nerve near the carotid artery. That slowed his heart rate and decreased the blood flow to his brain. When he moved his head again, the pressure on the nerve eased and his heart started racing to compensate for the drop in blood flow.

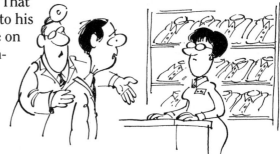

John, who wrote about the incidents in the *Philadelphia Inquirer* magazine, chucked his 15½-inch collars for new shirts with 16½-inch collars. He hasn't had a fainting spell since.

Get That Sucker Out of Here!

In 1989, a women went to the emergency room in Syracuse, New York, complaining that a cockroach was stuck in her ear.

Dr. Leo Rotello promptly shot a squirt of lidocaine into her ear and waited for the bug to crawl out. But the cockroach stayed put. So Dr. Rotello sprayed another dose of lidocaine into her ear. The bug still wouldn't budge.

By now, the woman was screaming. While Dr. Rotello was consulting with another physician over what to do, the now-hysterical patient screamed, "Get that sucker out of here!"

What a good idea, thought Dr. Rotello. He reached for a suction device on the wall which normally was used to suck up excess liquid spills. He inserted the tip of the device into the woman's ear and sucked out the cockroach in no time at all.

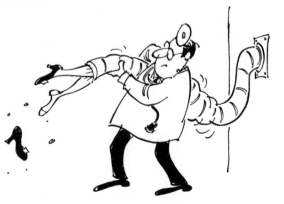

99

A Bitter Bill to Swallow

Dr. Roland Cross of Loyola Medical College in Chicago received the strangest bill of his life in 1986.

The statement said he owed $309 for anesthesia during the recent Caesarean delivery that he had undergone.

The amused physician called the accounting department and informed them that he had not been hospitalized for any reason in his adult life. Besides, a seventy-year-old male like him would not be having a C-section without creating quite a stir throughout the world. And there had been no stir that he was aware of.

The hospital apologized and blamed the mistake on its computer. Dr. Cross figured that would be the last of it.

He was wrong.

Several weeks later, he received a letter from Blue Cross stating that his hospital bill had been paid—for $309 for anesthesia during his Caesarean delivery. Not only that, but Blue Cross further offered its congratulations—on the birth of his twins!

Woman Bills Doctor for Long Wait

A woman was so fed up after sitting two hours in the waiting room of a physician that she billed him for her wasted time.

And, amazingly, he agreed to pay!

In 1995, Harriet Runyon of Scottsdale, Arizona, escorted an elderly uncle on a visit to the eye doctor. As they waited and waited long after the appointment, Harriet fumed and fumed.

"When we finally saw the doctor, he didn't offer any explanation or apology," she later told a reporter.

So when Harriet returned home, she acted on her anger. Figuring her time was worth fifty dollars an hour, she fired off a bill to the doctor for one hundred dollars.

The stunned doctor later called her and wanted to know how she could think her time was so valuable. Harriet replied that she had just received a bill from him for eight hundred dollars for a procedure that had taken only twenty minutes.

The doctor took Harriet's argument to heart and deducted one hundred dollars from the bill to compensate her for the time she wasted in his waiting room.

Where There's a Will There's a Way

As a nurse, Maria Rodriguez had seen enough patients and their families suffer when lives were prolonged by artificial means.

"I would never want my family to suffer seeing me in a vegetative state, to have them mortgage their homes and go broke paying for my care," she told the press.

So in 1995 the forty-year-old nurse from Gary, Indiana, had a living will tattooed on her stomach.

The red and black tattoo featured a red heart slashed with the universal "no" sign and the words "No Code." The will reads: "Pain and comfort only. Organ donor." It ends with her initials, "M.R."

The "No Code" instructs hospital and ambulance workers not to resuscitate her or keep her alive by artificial means.

"When my name gets called, I don't want anything holding me up," she said.

Indiana's living will statute requires the will to be dated and signed by the person writing it along with two witnesses. Although her will doesn't meet those requirements, Maria said she hopes it is respected.

Medicine: When in good health, make fun of it.

— Gustave Flaubert, *nineteenth-century French writer*

Bus Driver Faints while Hearing Surgery Story

A squeamish bus driver became so ill as he listened to a passenger describe an operation in detail that he passed out at the wheel. The bus then plowed into eight parked cars.

Details of the bizarre 1993 accident were revealed in court in Liverpool, England.

Bus driver Michael Lount, who testified he can't stand the sight of blood, said that he became queasy when a woman passenger launched into a graphic account of her recent hysterectomy. Her surgical story caused him to faint before he could step on the brakes.

Nevertheless, the judge put the blame for the crash on the driver—ruling that Lount should simply not have listened to the unpleasant account while driving a crowded bus. The bus company was ordered to pay damages to the owners of the cars that were struck.

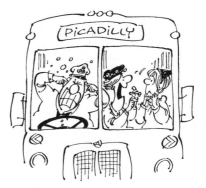

Bearers of Bad Tidings

A determined ambulance crew arrived at the address, forced the man onto a stretcher, strapped him down, ignored his objections, and rushed him to the hospital.

Only then did the crew realize their man had a legitimate beef. This guy was healthy—and angry. That's because they had gone to the wrong house and picked up the wrong guy!

In describing the mix-up, which occurred in 1995 in Norway, the forty-four-year-old man told the Oslo newspaper *Verdens Gang,* "I tried to protest when the ambulance came. But then I was told that from then on they were making the decisions and that I had no say in it."

The ambulance crew was supposed to pick up an ailing fifty-seven-year-old. But they got confused. Both he and the wrong man had the same name, lived in the same village, and had been to the same hospital for tests.

When the ambulance failed to show for the sick man, he managed to drive himself nearly forty miles to the hospital in the south Norway town of Kragero. When he arrived, the hospital at first refused to admit him. The clerk insisted the poor fellow was already there!